Fat Doctor Thin Doctor Series

LEAN ON ME

YOUR JOURNEY TO FOREVER THIN

ISBN 978-0-9968890-0-1

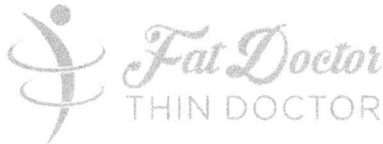

Fat Doctor
THIN DOCTOR

TABLE OF CONTENTS

INTRODUCTION

Obesity is the major health issue of our time. Eighty percent of Americans are overweight. You already know this. The key question you are asking yourself is how can I lose the excess fat and live life at my optimal weight? I have great news. Anyone who suffers from obesity or being overweight can conquer this disease. It is critical to understand the problem and why you find it so difficult to lose the weight and to keep it off over the long term. It is a complex disorder, but you can beat it once and for all. The answer is not a new 15 minute a day program, or a 30 day challenge. Nor is it a new machine or a supplement sold on late night TV. It is not due to a lack of discipline or willpower. The answers to this disease and this dilemma are well-known. I have used them for myself and thousands of my patients on our journey to thin. I want to share these answers and a specific map with you. I will walk with you on your journey to forever thin.

I was a Fat Doctor. It sounds like two words that shouldn't be found together. Don't doctors know all about health and getting healthy? Don't doctors learn about nutrition, exercise, human physiology, and how to maintain their health when they go through medical school? Don't they know how to help their patients lose weight and to maintain the weight loss? If doctors know how to combat weight problems and obesity, then why is America and the rest of the world getting fatter every year? These are great questions!

It's true that I was a Fat Doctor. One of my patients called me out on it. I will talk more about my story later. Some physicians have only recently decided that obesity is an actual disease. A committee of renowned doctors debated this point and voted to determine if obesity should be classified as a medical disease. It passed by only one vote. The minority opinion was that obesity is not a disease. It is well-known that obesity can cause many diseases such as hypertension, diabetes, arthritis, heart disease, certain cancers, and many others. These diseases can also exist without the presence of obesity, but significant excess body fat will dramatically increase the likelihood of their occurrence.

Over the last 14 years of my career in Family Medicine, my practice has focused on the problem of obesity. I have studied many theories and ideas about the reasons for the U.S. obesity epidemic. I have attended numerous educational conferences, obesity symposia, nutritional meetings and read everything I could get my hands on regarding the management of food and fat. I have worked closely with my own obese and overweight patients since 2001. I have not only been the treating physician, but also the patient. Through this focus of study and the daily practice of evaluating, diagnosing, and treating patients with weight issues and the resultant negative health effects, I have gained a greater understanding of the problems, treatments, and obstacles that my patients and I face every day on the journey to getting leaner and staying thinner.

Do we need another book on obesity? Many will argue that we don't, but to date the problems of excess fat gain and obesity are not getting better, they are getting worse. If a cure for obesity was available at this time, we would all be thin. Earlier this year, some statistics came out claiming that childhood obesity is showing a slowdown in growth. I suspect these statistics are true, but may be similar to reported statistics showing a slowdown in government spending. Statistics can be a funny thing. They can be factual and misleading at the same time. In our practice, we still see an amazing number of children with obesity and even Type II Diabetes. Nonetheless, obesity is rampant and its brother disease of Type II Diabetes is growing at alarming rates in the United States. Until we address the true causes of obesity and the solutions to this devastating health problem, new ideas and information can only move us in a positive direction in finding an answer for anyone and everyone that bears the burden of being fat. I'm presenting my ideas to you through this book. I hope they lead to remission and long term control of your weight disorder.

I use the terms "Fat" and "Obesity" readily and often. Some of my patients have been offended by my use of these terms. I feel that hiding the problem under terminology like "large framed", "full figured", "big boned", and "ample" are just ways of softening the connotation of being fat in our society and is an attempt at being more politically correct than honest. When my patient said "Doc, you're fat", she was right. When I stood on the scales and calculated my Body Mass Index, I looked at myself in the mirror and agreed by uttering, "I'm fat". Being fat and ignoring it is dangerous. Being fat and getting help in figuring out how to beat it is powerful and can change your life for the better, forever. As you read along, don't be offended by these terms. They are true and certainly much easier to write and read than the softer alternatives. If you have a Body Mass Index over 30, you are obese. If your Body Mass Index (BMI) is above 24 and under 30, you are overweight. We'll look at BMI later on and go over why it's not the best measurement to determine your health, but it is a good starting point. So, if you are above your ideal weight range, accept it and let's move on to work together to make you a leaner, fitter, healthier you.

My purpose in writing this book is to let you know that no matter how many diets, programs, trainers, meetings, and weight loss "miracles" you have been through or tried, there is still hope and an answer for you. Even if you've read all the books in the weight loss section at the bookstore, I will give you new information that will show you that you can become the size and the person you know exists in your currently overweight body. Information in itself will never solve a problem. Acting on the information is where the solution lies. I have patients, who during our first meeting say, "I just can't lose the weight". They, like most people struggling with excess body fat, have been through the gamut of commercial programs, every new weight loss fad and supplement, and the yo-yo of losing 20 pounds and gaining it back over and over. Another reason for this book is to let you know that you are not alone. Yes, I realize that everywhere you look there are many obese people and many who are larger than you; but, you like most of the others feel that there is something specifically wrong with yourself that keeps you from dropping the pounds and the fat.

When you are finished with this book, you will have a greater understanding of why you are overweight, what can be done about it, and how to take reasonable and consistent steps to become a healthier, thinner, more energetic individual ready to take on the world and not spend every day thinking about your weight. At this point, you may feel like a chronic dieter and that this is your life's health path, but just like everything else in life you can take command of this issue and conquer it once and for all. It will take focus. It will take hard work, and it will take the attitude of a professional. We all know that professionals in every field rise above the rest. Professional athletes are the absolute best in their sport. They make up much less than 1% of people who ever played their sport. Professionals in medicine, finance, law, teaching, and engineering are the best of the best. We call many people professionals, but only a very small number are truly in this category.

Are you a professional when it comes to health and the achievement of your optimal weight? Probably not, but you can become one. I know that it sounds weird that we can become a professional or pro in weight loss and weight maintenance. Only about 5% of people who lose significant weight will maintain the loss for greater than 5 years. These are the professionals at weight loss and maintenance. They do things that the rest of people who lose and gain, lose and gain, over and over fail to do. If you knew what these pro's do, would you commit to doing it? I suspect that you would say yes. Saying yes and doing the work are two different things. However,

I plan to help you become a pro in this endeavor. You can do every one of the things that the pros do. You are about to embark on a life changing journey that will create the health and the life you want. When you are at your lean and healthy weight you will live a life that many desire and all can achieve, yet few actually do. Let's get started on the quest for a lean, fit, strong and healthy body and a vibrant, exciting and long life.

It's time to stop looking at the weight loss process as something we "have to do" and begin to see it as something we "get to do". We get to be thin, we get to be fit, and we get to be healthy. These are not things that only some people can achieve. Every person can achieve a leaner, fitter, stronger, and healthy body. Anybody can chose to be thin and commit to the treatment of obesity. The journey to thin follows a specific map that I will present to you. By staying on the correct path and following this map, you will reach and maintain your best weight. It can be an exciting process and adventure. Changing our lives for the better is always exciting. You will focus on the outcome and not get bogged down by the process. The process will become habit and the positive results will drive you to live in the body you've wanted but thought was unattainable. Feel free to LEAN on me during your journey to thin.

If you need someone to scream at, scream at me. If you need someone to swear at, swear at me. If you need encouragement or a pat on the back, I'll be happy to assist. If you need a coach or an accountability partner, count on me. My goal is to help you become a thinner, more energetic, healthy person that can do everything you to do and get the most out of your life. Fat Doctor / Thin Doctor is just the beginning of our journey together. Let's get started on our journey to Forever Thin.

CHAPTER 1
OBESITY—THE PERFECT STORM

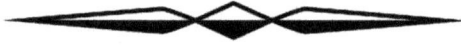

To understand and undertake the journey to thin, awareness and knowledge of the problem that has created too much fat in our body is critical. You can't read a newspaper, magazine, or see a news show without someone talking about the epidemic of obesity in America and its spread throughout the world. There are specific reasons why humans are getting fatter which doesn't have to do with laziness and gluttony (at least in most cases). Discipline is an important factor, but only a small part of the problem. Willpower plays a role, but again only a small role. Without understanding the problem, solving it will be impossible. Obesity rates have only grown dramatically since the mid 1970's. Before that decade, obesity rates were always somewhat low and steady. What happened in the 1970's that started the rapid and accelerating rates of obesity? Let's explore these reasons and the multiple factors that have made it much easier for humans to gain weight more easily and why losing weight has become much more difficult for each overweight individual. Knowing these reasons will assist you as you undertake this exciting journey to become lean.

The first and most important fact about obesity is that we as humans were made to make and store fat. Without this ability, our ancestors would not have survived on earth long enough for us to be here today. Our distant ancestors spent their entire lives in search of their meals. From the time the sun rose until it set and at times throughout the night, they searched for food. Massive amounts of energy were expended to get a meal. They hiked, climbed, dug, chased, and fought to get their food. When a meal was found or killed, they would eat the entirety of the food as no storage system was available. They would overeat and their bodies would make fat from the excess food and this would sustain them until their next meal; or, until they moved on to a location with more food; or, until the season changed and food was more plentiful. Those that could make and store fat the best, had the greatest chance of survival and living long enough to have children to carry on. The genetics of the survivors were passed on and each generation became more efficient at processing food into energy and storing fat for needed energy in lean times. We are the inheritors of these fat producing, fat storing genetics. We are ultra-efficient fat formers. We have "Fat Genes"!

Knowing that our bodies are great at making and storing fat, let's look at what changed in the 1970's. Our western culture was now in full transition from the industrial age to the information age. Technology was advancing rapidly with the advent of computing machines. The science of the NASA space missions and moon missions was filtering into our daily lives. Every home had modern conveniences which were getting better, faster, and more efficient each year. Television was now firmly entrenched in nearly every home in America. Comfort and convenience was the name of the game for marketers and manufacturers. As life became more comfortable and less energy was needed to be expended to perform daily tasks, our need to store fat for energy decreased. Populations were moving from the farms to the cities. As we moved through the 1980's and 1990's, the trend continued with more remote controls, push button devices, and less and less manual effort needed to get through the day. Jobs that required physical labor were decreasing in number with many jobs being sent to countries where labor costs were lower than in the United States. Service jobs and desk jobs were the growing sectors of our work force. The number of women who stayed at home to care for children was decreasing and these women entered the work force initially in clerical and support roles spending

8 or more hours daily in their seats at the companies they worked for. The beginning of the 21ˢᵗ century saw an exponential expansion of the computer age with devices that made our work and lives easier, but took away the need to perform physical labor. School programs were dropping their physical education programs and only those kids who played sports were getting adequate exercise. The overall trend was less human energy expenditure and more machine and robot energy expenditure.

During this same period of time, beginning after World War II, agricultural science and technology was moving in the same direction with greater production of genetically modified plants and animals allowing for higher yields in food production to feed the planet and less laborers to produce the food. Machinery and technology had made the small family farm obsolete and large corporate farms facilitated vast food production without the need for many workers. Food was becoming more calorie dense and the level of carbohydrates in our diet was rapidly rising. Processing of foods into new and innovative products was rampant. Foods that now came in a bag were everywhere and a new variety of snacks was seen almost every month. New foods like the Twinkie, Ding Dong, any type of soda, and every possible chip and cracker was available. Fast food which began in the 1940's and 1950's was being franchised and duplicated so that every person in America could have it readily available. We could now drive up to a restaurant, push the automatic window button in our car and 2000 calories was passed through without the need to hardly use a muscle. Food taste and food marketing was being perfected so that Americans were now being told what to eat from the TV while sitting on the most comfortable chair in the world, the recliner. A new term was coined, "the Couch Potato".

During this same time period (1992), the U.S. Government was working to let us know what foods were good for us through the use of their version of the "Official Food Guide Pyramid". This Guide advised us to eat low fat and to make sure the foundation of our diet was 6–11 servings of carbohydrates (grain based foods) daily. Because the government said it was good for us, dietitians were taught this, school lunch programs complied, and even the medical community jumped on board. As Americans became fatter and fatter, they were told that they were just eating too much and that they were not disciplined in their eating and activity behavior. Americans felt guilty that something was wrong with them as individuals. We were being taught to eat the wrong types and amounts of food.

Daily stress was now a part of the nature of our work and our play. Working longer hours and taking work home was the way to the top of the corporate ladder. Keeping up with the neighbors by borrowing more to have the best house, best car, best clothes and newest gadgets was an obsession. Our kids had to be in the best schools and be on every team and go to every event. As a result, we were living each day as if it had 36 hours instead of 24. This stress that we put on ourselves led the body to respond by producing excess amounts of cortisol and adrenaline which over time have an adverse effect on our ability to process and utilize foods properly. More fat was being produced in our body due to the mental and physical stress on our bodies. With more work, more stress, and the rapid expansion of television technology and programming, we were also now sleeping less. Less sleep leads to hormonal alteration and the resultant faulty appetite signaling and food processing mechanisms in the body. The ability to gain fat and the difficulty in losing fat was now well established in nearly 80% of the population by the end of the first decade of the 2000's.

Another factor in the escalation of obesity in our society has been more recently found to be the stimulation of our brains by foods high in sugar. Receptors in the eating centers of our brain respond to the sugar and create the desire for eating additional sugar or sweets. Even non-caloric sweeteners have been thought to produce increased eating behavior through this mechanism. The D2 dopamine receptor in the brain has been found to be a factor in excess sugar and sweet intake and with excess eating and craving behavior. This same receptor is found to be a major player in people with dependency on known addictive substances such as nicotine, cocaine, and narcotics. I tell many of my patients that experience the inability to stop eating sweets and sugar-based foods, that they most likely have developed a "soft addiction" to sugar. The only reason I call it a "soft addiction" is that these patients will not have seizures or dramatic withdrawal symptoms like they might from withdrawal from the other addictive substances. These patients who are sensitive to sugars tell me that they intellectually and logically understand that they should stop eating the sweet foods, but at the same time continue to put them in their mouth. There are now over 2700 published peer reviewed journal articles and books in the medical literature that deal with the physical craving of food and with the chemical dependency we develop to foods.

The perfect storm leading to the modern obesity epidemic is the gathering of these multiple factors I have discussed, including our genetics, current work pattern, technology, food science leading to a dietary change, faulty theory on healthy diet, diminished exercise and activity requirements, and biochemical changes in our bodies in response to this diet, stress, and sleep pattern changes. The newer science of food addiction and physical craving mechanisms, I believe, will ultimately show that most obese patients will require medical, psychological, and therapeutic intervention to allow for significant weight loss and the maintenance of a lower, healthier body weight. This confluence of factors in the Obesity Perfect Storm will need to be evaluated for each obese patient and a specific individual treatment plan established if long term control of overeating and obesity treatment is to be successful. There is no cookie-cutter answer to the disease of obesity. Certainly discipline and will-power play a role, but these are not the primary culprits of serious weight gain and obesity.

Knowing that there are some factors not of our doing that have allowed for excess fat and weight gain don't let us off the hook for taking charge of our lives and working to move toward a leaner and much healthier body size. Being overweight is not your fault, but treating and managing the problem for improved health is your responsibility. It should give us hope that we can grasp the issues that lead to our obesity and allow us to establish a plan of treatment to correct the condition. We are always responsible for ourselves. Our health, fitness, body size and composition are our responsibility. Being responsible means that what I think, do, and how I do it are up to me. I can't control if another person on the road pulls out in front of me and causes an accident. I am still responsible for having made the decision to drive, whether I have adequate insurance, and how I respond to the incident. The same is true with regard to our health. We didn't get to pick our genes or our parents. We didn't get to choose where we were born and where we lived, but we do get to decide what we do about it. We can decide to make the effort to learn all we can about our bodies and our current state of health. We can decide if we are going to take action to work on reducing the fat content of our bodies and we can choose if we are going to be consistent and committed to the weight loss program. All I'm saying is that we can't control the cards we were dealt, but we can decide how we play them. My goal is to show you how to play the cards in the best way possible to get the results you are wanting to achieve in getting to your goal weight and improved level of health. I know that you can live lean, live long, and live life to the fullest. Take charge now! Choose thin and choose health. These choices are exciting and can drive you to your vision of a fit and trim body.

CHAPTER 2
PERSONAL PAIN AND THE WAR WITHIN US

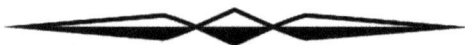

I want to be at my ideal weight today and I don't want to have to do anything to get there. I don't understand why some people can eat anything they want and not gain weight and I gain weight just looking at food. I don't want to have to think about food, my diet, exercising, and tracking all of this every day of my life. I just want to be thin and over this whole weight issue. Have you ever thought any of these thoughts to yourself? I know you have because these are the things I've thought about and all of my patients acknowledge to me on a regular basis. We blame ourselves and think that for some reason we just don't have the willpower or the discipline to stay on a healthy eating plan and get a bit more physical activity every day. Society tells us we're just lazy and that if we just eat less and exercise more we'll be thin. Hollywood lets us know all the time that we are imperfect and no matter what we do we will never look like the stars on TV or the Big Screen.

Our excess weight haunts us every day. We look for clothes that will hide the extra bulge. We avoid situations that will expose the real us. We don't want to go to the pool or the beach and those high school reunions . . . who wants to go and see people we haven't seen in years anyway. The last thing we want now is for anyone with a cell phone camera snapping our pics every time we turn around. I don't need my overweight body showing up on your Facebook page. Carrying the unwanted pounds consumes our thoughts. We think about food. We think about eating. We plan our day around eating, and eventually we eat too much food and then obsess about overeating and gaining additional weight. In more extreme cases, we hide our eating habits and become closet eaters to avoid eating around others. Being overweight or obese has a negative stigma attached to it and almost everyone that carries the extra weight also carries the internal strife of living in their oversized body. We can laugh at ourselves, we can belittle ourselves, we can ignore ourselves, and we can hide from ourselves, but no matter what we do, inside we feel a sense of frustration, shame, and pain. Being overweight or obese certainly does not diminish anyone as a person and should never overshadow the wonderful qualities of each individual. However, we are typically our own harshest critics and if others won't harass us over our weight, we will certainly become the lead perpetrator of our own personal mental beatings.

The pain of being fat comes from our internal feeling that we have done something wrong and that our obesity is the result of our own weakness. On one hand, we savor the taste of a sweet treat, and then moments later admonish ourselves for having eaten it. Our minds are conflicted. We say we want to be thinner and healthier, but we regret each and every meal we eat especially if it wasn't the best choice we could have made. Over time, the constant internal nagging at ourselves gives way to a sense of hopelessness and for many the acceptance that "this is just the way I'm supposed to be". I will suffer the ill health, physical constraints and personal defeat and go on with my life to the best of my ability. This negative internal dialogue plays over and over inside the mind of the obese person. Negative thinking creates a downward vicious cycle and feeds on itself until we feel that we are the reason for our obesity and that in some odd way we deserve to be fat. Breaking this negative thought cycle is critical to overcoming obesity. Obesity is a condition and a disorder. Our environment and food choices play a big role, but I've yet to meet an obese person who set off on a goal to get fat. Anyone who has done that is dealing with a different and more significant emotional disorder and needs psychological counseling.

The pain of obesity is insidious. Overeating and gaining weight occurs slowly and therefore is only recognized by each of us once we are already have added significant extra pounds of fat. We usually only begin to fret when someone else calls it to our attention, or when on a shopping spree we notice the clothes we thought we could wear no longer fit. Recognition of our excess fat occurs when we stop for a moment and actually take a hard look at ourselves in the mirror. Our minds tend to ignore the gaining of weight until it becomes noticeable in one of these ways. Our mind wants to protect us from the realization that we are actually hurting ourselves. This is seen with smokers, who seem to be totally oblivious to the ill effects on their health, even though the warnings are everywhere, even on the cigarette pack. The pain of realizing we are actually dangerous to our own survival is too painful for our mind to focus on and therefore this pain is suppressed into some dark recess of our brain.

Carrying significant extra fat will shorten our lives, reduce our energy level, cause a domino effect of future diseases, lower our self-esteem, reduce success in the work environment, diminish sexual desire and function, and cause many more negative daily issues. Even with all of these negative effects, the delay in taking action to combat this disorder is universal. All of us dieters know that each and every program or plan we've been on works well, at first, and then the weight loss slows and reversal occurs over time. It seems to us that it's the rare person who loses the weight and keeps it off. Remembering our failed weight loss experiences, leads us into avoidance of taking on the task again. We become conditioned to avoid the pain of weight loss, but at the same time hate the pain of obesity.

Pain of obesity and pain of not accomplishing our long term goals with regard to our weight become major players in the ongoing conflict in the mind of the overweight. The internal talk of "I need to lose this weight", and "I've tried and failed at it many times before" banter back and forth. For the stress eaters, this internal strife aggravates the eating problem and leads to additional weight gain. If you are someone who has experienced this frustrating emotional battle, there is great hope for you. We have a remarkable capacity to change our thinking. We can take control of our brain by using our mind. The way we think can actually change the patterns running in our brain. In order to beat the weight loss / weight gain cycle, we must change not only our eating patterns and our activity patterns, but also our thinking patterns. I will teach you as we go along how to get control of all three of these success patterns. It is possible to conquer the obesity problem even knowing that your weight gain and excess body fat are caused by many factors that are out of our control. You can beat the genetics, biochemistry, and environmental factors. I am going to partner with you on beating the obesity disorder. We will move together toward a mind and body that is focused on maintaining a lean weight and living a lean life full of energy. Eliminating the daily physical and emotional pain of obesity is my goal for you. It is possible to learn how to successfully approach the problem and to take a worthwhile and exhilarating journey. We will move forward and beat Obesity together.

CHAPTER 3
FAT DOCTOR/THIN DOCTOR—MY LESSONS AND YOUR VICTORY

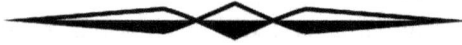

Being a practicing family physician should give me some credibility in assisting you with reaching your weight loss goal. Unfortunately, many very good family physicians, internists, ob-gyn physicians, and other specialists are either ill prepared to manage the disease of obesity or feel that it is not their responsibility. Treating the diseases associated with obesity becomes the focus of most primary care and specialty practices. Only when diabetes is rampant, blood pressure and cholesterol are uncontrolled, and symptoms of heart disease arise are doctors called into action to treat the patient. Unfortunately, when symptoms occur or the numbers are bad, the disease is not at its beginning phase, but in its later stages.

In the past, treating obesity was viewed by the medical community as being on the fringe and definitely not science based. It was felt that the few doctors that did run weight loss clinics were just in it for the money and their practices were dangerous and bordered on quackery. Over the past decade, many good and caring physicians have entered the new field of Bariatric Medicine. Specialty boards are now forming with specific educational requirements. Large national and international conferences and meetings on obesity, its causes, treatment and management are now common. Thousands of medical studies have been done on weight gain, appetite, and factors that create obesity. Research into obesity is going on at a fever pitch. Realizing that if the obesity epidemic is not contained and reversed, our healthcare system will fail. This has motivated some individuals to start taking a closer look at the causes and treatment of this devastating disease. With this revelation, medicine and science are now moving in the proper direction of assisting patients with weight loss and improved health through prevention of disease. I woke up to this problem one afternoon in 2001.

I became interested in helping my patients lose weight in the early 2000's. One day, I was seeing patients in my office. My first patient after my lunch break was a wonderful little lady in her late 70's named Natalie. I had known her for years, but today when I entered the exam room and said hello, she looked me over and said, "Doc, You're Fat!" I was taken back, embarrassed and a bit shocked. However, she was right. My BMI had climbed above 30 and that made me obese. After taking care of Natalie's medical problem, I moved on to my other patients that day, but circling in my mind was the nagging thought that Natalie had planted. "I'm Fat". I was telling my patients to lose weight, eat less, and exercise more and was handing out diet sheets. However, I had not even realized that my own weight had shot up to 225 pounds. I had always been athletic in high school and college and typically stayed near my ideal weight of 175 pounds. The usual things happened to me as with most of my patients. I became focused on my family and my career. I no longer thought that I had the time to dedicate to eating right and exercising. With a family history of obesity and easy weight gain along with a strong desire for carbohydrates and sweets, the pounds piled on. My visit with Natalie was an eye opener for me, not just personally, but professionally.

I decided that for both my and my patient's benefit, I would start to learn about obesity. I wanted to know if it was just due to overeating and lack of activity, or whether there were certain factors that made this a more complex problem. Eating less and exercising more was what I had been asking my patients to do to lose weight. It wasn't working for them either. It seemed like only a rare patient ever lost a significant amount of weight. Of course, we all know that eating less and exercising more will result in weight and fat loss. However, if that is true then why was it so difficult for me and my patients to drop weight and keep it off? I felt that there had to be other factors. I began my educational journey into the disorder of obesity. After attending conferences and extensive reading and studying, I developed my own weight loss program. Within 3 ½ months, I was back at my goal weight in the 170's. Though eating less and exercising more is a simple concept, I found that it was not easy. It did seem to matter what types of foods I ate, and what schedule and type of exercise I performed. Being able to control my thinking and my emotional perspective of food was the most difficult part.

I soon learned that willpower was only a small part of the formula. Before this weight loss undertaking, I thought it was all about willpower and discipline. I didn't have a lack of willpower or discipline. I had graduated from high school, college, medical school and developed a medical practice. This took a tremendous amount of willpower and discipline. Each of my patients demonstrated this same willpower operating in their lives. They had used their discipline to finish school, get work, hold onto a job or business, raise a family, and all of the things that life requires of us. Why did it seem like willpower went out the window for everyone when it came to weight loss? Willpower and discipline are necessary for weight loss, but they are not the most important things by a long shot. This is great news for us weight losers. I am going to teach and share with you the current theories, science, treatments, and information about weight loss and weight management that I learned along my journey to thin. I will share with you how to overcome setbacks and struggles and how to turn the path to getting lean into an enjoyable experience. I learned so much about this disease (as well as about myself and my patients) that I wanted to share with you how to become forever thin.

My trip to lean seemed quick and easy to anyone who just saw the 45+ pounds disappear over a few months. That was not true. I had daily struggles and setbacks and felt like giving up at least once a day. Upon reaching my target weight, I realized that the real work was just beginning. As always in life, stuff happens. I remained lean for the next few years with a focused effort and a routine of healthy eating and regular physical activity. Then a crazy thing happened on the journey to stay thin. Every one of my patients who is on a program or plan of ours goes through crazy times and crazy distractions. It almost seems that the day we decide to lose weight and get healthy, the minions of distraction and interference attack us. I've heard from my patients everything in the book that has tried to shift them off of the path to getting healthy. Many could call these excuses, but it is real life stuff requiring focus and attention that comes into everyone's life. Learning to overcome these distractions and to persist with a healthy eating and activity pattern in the face of adversity or stress is the most important thing than can be learned from the arrival of life's unexpected events.

My event occurred one day in my office when I suddenly felt a strange sensation in my chest and a bit of weakness. As a physician, I knew right away that I was having a cardiac dysrhythmia (heart irregular rhythm). I called my nurse into the room to get an EKG test and found I was in a rhythm called Atrial Fibrillation. Of course, I didn't treat myself, although I wanted to. Instead, sought the assistance of a cardiology colleague. Over the next seven years, I was prescribed several medications to attempt to control the recurrence of the disorder, none of which worked. These medications were heart rhythm calming agents with the potential for many side effects. I got many of the side effects, the worst of which was a 25 pound weight gain. I couldn't exercise because each time I did, I went into Atrial Fibrillation. I found it increasingly difficult to keep my weight down with this heart irregularity, the medication side effects, and my inability to be active. I felt bad in my weight loss clinic talking to patients about all of the things they should be doing to control their weight and not being able to personally do them myself. I did continue eating healthy, but without much movement. With my heart rate and blood pressure at severely low levels on the meds, I felt like sitting or sleeping most of the time. New treatments for A-Fib were being developed during this period. My goal was to get the problem resolved and not just manage it, which wasn't working anyway. I had gone from having an episode of A-Fib every few months to several episodes a week and was heading for persistent daily Atrial Fibrillation and permanent medication therapy. I went to several cardiologists and was able to get on the schedule for a cardiac ablation treatment to try to eliminate the rhythm. Essentially, they put probes into the heart and attempted to burn electrical pathways to eliminate the abnormal rhythm. After 7.5 hours in the procedure room, I was hopeful to get back to my original active self and get these 25 pounds off. After these procedures, there is a healing period and success can only be determined after 3–6 months. Fortunately, I had no further Atrial Fibrillation and was able to get off all of the medications and find my old self again.

Within a short period of time, I had lost 18 pounds and decided that it was time to get to my target weight again. The reason I am recounting this story to you is to let you know that life is not always simple. When we are focused on losing weight and staying at a healthy weight, things happen. Many of these things are not in our control. Loss of a job, financial issues, illness or death in a family, children problems, and more issues than I could ever list will confront us throughout our lives. Just like my sudden and prolonged heart disorder that came on for no apparent reason, you too will have events and distractions that affect you. Some of the issues you confront may actually be detrimental to losing weight such as being placed on a medication for another health reason. No matter what comes our way, learning to face the issue head on and figuring out how to deal with it in a manner that doesn't move us from our original vision of our lives and our goals is the key to a successful life.

Everyone has problems. Everyone has to deal with these problems. Being able to live in the solution rather than living in the problem will change your life. It will change every aspect of your life for the positive. Learning to handle stress in a more constructive way will also contribute to a healthier body. Lowering stress also has a positive effect on our weight. Less stress (or handling it better) lowers production of the stress hormone cortisol. Cortisol promotes fat production in our body. Stress will come. How you manage it and deal with it can either wreck your mind and body or can take you to living at a much higher and improved level. We get to choose. These are some of the lessons I have learned on my journey to thin. Instead of frustration, I see fascination. Instead of problems, I see challenges. Instead of living in the problem, I live in the solution. I'm by no means perfect and my mind resists looking at things in this way, but my goal is to overcome complaining and excuse making and to take charge of my life. You can take charge of your life, no matter how bad things seem or whatever comes your way. By getting better at taking this responsibility, you will be able to take charge of your body and beat the genetics, the biochemistry and hormone issues, the environment of high calorie food on every street corner, and the patterns of bad personal choices that many times come from the erroneous meanings we place on our food. You will take charge of your body, your mind, and your personal environment to become the leaner, stronger, healthier person you were designed to be. My story is only an example of how deciding to lose weight and get lean can sound simple, but is a life long journey of combating the many causes of obesity and the crazy things that happen to us on our way to thin. Moving from overeater to overcomer is the objective you will undertake in order to arrive at your perfect weight. Your perfect weight is where you will feel, look, and be your best. I want to hear your story of how you overcame Resistance and adversity on your journey to thin.

CHAPTER 4
UNDERSTANDING THE ENEMY

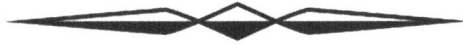

ANCESTRY

The human body was built for a time much different than today. We were created to evolve and change with our environment and the times. However, the ability for our bodies and minds to change is much slower than the change we create in our world. Our distant ancestors were made to make fat. To eat they had to hunt and chase their food. They had to climb, dig, forage, and move to get a meal. When they killed an animal or found a place rich in edibles, they would gorge themselves on the food and their bodies would make fat to store as energy until the next meal could be caught or found. Another meal might be a few days or longer away. It was a matter of survival that the body be able to store enough fuel to survive between meals.

Moving forward to today, the ability to store fat to protect us from starvation is not as important for our survival as it was to our ancestors. Food is plentiful. Food is relatively inexpensive. Food comes in thousands of configurations with multitudes of taste and variety. Food can be found in America on nearly every street at a mega-store, grocery, market, drive-thru, and even at every gas station. Because of the easy availability of food, our body's fat stores are rarely used as a primary energy source. We continue to make fat anytime we eat more than our body can utilize between meals. Over time, our body composition can become 30%, 50%, and in some cases even a greater percentage of fat. Normal fat percentages should never reach more than 25% fat. Very healthy fat percentages are in the teens or lower. Having some fat is critical to the health of our body, but excess fat actually has a detrimental effect. Our ancestors were much leaner than us. Their diets were also much different than ours. Their foods were much less likely to produce excess fat. Our current diets are high in grain based foods which are carbohydrates, and simple sugars. Our bodies are only able to utilize small amounts of these foods at a time. Any excesses are rapidly converted into fat for storage. Eating three meals a day and intermittent snacking provides many more calories than we can utilize.

Our current lifestyles are very sedentary compared with the life of our distant ancestors. They would walk, wander, and move about for days. No modern conveniences existed, so all of their efforts required personal physical labor. Our entire society is set up around making life more and more convenient for us. More convenience creates less physical activity which requires less food for fuel. Our ancestors lived on fish, wild vegetables, and fruits and nuts. Meats came to the menu later. The carbohydrates they ate had low amounts of sugars and were all natural and fiber filled. Only after agriculture techniques were developed, did we start to create foods that were more concentrated in calories and sugar. After the processing of foods began, the caloric content become denser and the level of sugar in the foods rose. Once humans learned to manipulate the growth of our food and then process the foods to create different tastes and products, we began to become obese as a society. We can take lessons from our ancestors and go back to eating more natural foods and less calorie dense foods. We must always remember that every extra calorie that our body doesn't use is a calorie of fat that will be made and become extra mass. We must learn to eat for our time. Our ancestors passed their fat storing ability on to each successive generation. Those with the ability to store fat the best survived and passed their fat storing genetics on to their children. We have inherited the fat genes. To beat the fat genes, we must re-learn to eat less food volume and to be intentionally active every day.

GENETICS

We now know that the ability to more easily become fat is a polygenetic trait. There is not <u>one</u> "fat gene". There are genes that make us more likely to prefer sugar. There are genes that make us poor digesters of grains. There are genes that make us produce too much cholesterol. We have many thousands of genes and yet we still do not know what most of them do for us or to us. We don't know what turns each gene on or off and how much of an effect each gene has on us. Genetic science knowledge is expanding at exponential rates, but is still in its infancy. Almost every disease has a genetic component to it. The ability to acquire diabetes, heart disease, or cancer is based in genetics. If the genetics are present in the right quantity or quality, then environmental triggers can set the genetic dance in motion. An example of variable genetic expression is seen when someone smokes for 50 or 60 years and does not develop lung cancer, yet another person smokes for 20 years and dies in their 40's of this disease. I believe it has to do with the genetics of each individual and how those genes direct our immune system and our tissues to respond to the environment. Genes tell our bodies how to handle foods and nutrients. They are at the root of how and why our bodies look, act and respond in a certain way.

The question to be answered is "Are we able to overcome the genetic predisposition that we each have"? I think that in most cases the answer is . . . yes. There are some genetic disorders that are manifested at 100%, meaning if you have the genes, you will get the trait and if that trait is a disease, you will get it. Other genetic disorders may be 50% manifested. There are others at 25% and so on. Some may only manifest in combination with other genetics or with influence from our environment. Our environment includes everything that is around us. Air, water, food, chemicals, natural and synthetic substances, bacteria, viruses, parasites, plants, other animals etc. Our interaction with every other thing in our world will affect us in a positive or negative way and each of us may respond differently to the same agent. A person that weighs 500 pounds didn't set out to become 500 pounds. A combination of circumstances set the enormous weight gain in motion. A collection of strong fat producing genetics is present in this person. A propensity for high sugar and fatty processed foods lead to excitation of addiction centers in their brain. A home environment rich in calorie dense food, along with low promotion of physical activity as a child plus too much screen time stimulate fat accumulation. Negatively spiraling hormonal changes in the body perpetuate the production of fat for the development of morbid obesity. Each person's genetic makeup will either predispose them to fast and easy weight gain, slow weight gain, or resistance to weight gain. Along with the genetic propensity for weight gain, the other conditions cited above trigger the process that ultimately leads to obesity. We can't change our genetics but we can beat the fat genes by taking personal control of our environment to reverse the downward spiral and turn it in a positive spinning direction. Becoming aware of the many factors that lead to body fat accumulation is a starting point for long term weight loss and weight control.

BIOCHEMISTRY

Biochemistry is the living, active, and functional chemistry that goes on at all times in all cells and spaces of our bodies. It is programmed by our genetics but altered by our environment. The molecules and chemical components of our body generate every thought, movement, and adjustment of our tissues, organs, and cells. What we breathe, drink and eat, and how we live can alter the chemistry of our body. How we think can alter the chemistry of our brains. When we eat too much fat, too many carbs, or just too many calories, we unleash a chemical storm in our bodies that has to work overtime to return to equilibrium. The calories have to be burned or stored. The foods have to be processed whether they're good for us or bad for us. The leftovers and resultant waste products must be eliminated. All of this occurs through chemical processes. When we eat too much, we put these processes into overdrive and the results are excess toxins and excess stress on our vital functions. The stress on our physical tissues and organs is magnified as our body attempts to bring its internal workings back to a steady state of stability. As we gain excess fat tissue, our biochemistry changes. The excess fat itself is an organ and for many people it becomes the largest organ in their body. This organ of fat creates its own chemistry, much of which is toxic to our body. Alterations in our blood, cholesterols, and hormones occur. As a result, our body is constantly fighting and compensating for this attack from within. Eating healthy and choosing foods wisely and in the right volume will allow our chemistry to work at its normal pace. The waste products and toxins that are produced from all of the reactions occurring in the body can be processed and handled in a smooth and normal fashion.

It's now known that the ingestion of high concentrations of sugar will lead to overstimulation of the pleasure centers of our brain. These same pleasure centers can be stimulated by addictive drugs such as nicotine, cocaine, narcotics, and any other substance that can cause dependency. When this brain area receives high levels of sugar, receptors are stimulated and dopamine (the feel good chemical) is released. The brain wants more of this feel good substance and more sugar is taken in. We can logically think that we should stop eating the cookies and the candy, but the brain and its potent chemical excitation have other ideas. I have often desired a simple single chocolate chip cookie and by the end of the day the bag is empty. It's almost as if there is a second person in my brain. This is the power of chemistry and the alterations in our behavior that can result from making the unhealthy eating choices on a regular basis. I call this phenomenon of uncontrolled sugar binging, "carbohydrate sensitivity", or a "soft sugar addiction". Many of my patients in our weight loss clinic will recognize this behavior when I explain it to them. They state "I am a sugar addict". Add fat to the carbs and now we have a deadly concentration of brain chemistry alteration. The French fry and donut are prime examples of foods that call our name and when eaten start yelling loudly for us to devour more. We must learn to protect our body chemistry and to keep control of our brain chemistry. By finally learning to take charge of our biochemistry, we can reduce the fat accumulation in our body and reduce the toxins and inflammation levels that lead to disease. I will share how to take charge of your chemistry and allow your body to reach a state of health that will increase your energy, stamina, strength, and longevity. By learning to positively affect your own biochemistry, you can create health and beat the genetics that otherwise will map out a short life of obesity and its sibling disease states.

HORMONES

Hormones are a subset of our biochemistry. I believe that the malfunctioning of our hormones is the main determinant of obesity and excess fat gain. When I say hormones, most people think about the sex hormones like testosterone, estrogen, and progesterone. These are important in our overall health and do play a role in weight fluctuations and obesity. However, other hormones play a more significant role in abnormal weight gain. Insulin is a hormone that plays a major role in the management of our fuel sources. Glucose (sugar) and Ketones (from fat) are the two fuels that our body uses. Our bodies prefer sugar because it's simpler and more efficient to burn. The brain can only burn these two fuels and prefers to burn sugar as its primary energy source. By adjusting our diet, we can re-direct our body to burn different ratios of glucose and fat. When we lower our glucose or carbohydrate intake and increase our protein intake but keep our overall calorie intake below our daily needs, we can shift the body into a fat burning mode. Insulin's opposite hormone is known as glucagon which goes to work in our body to shift to using our fat stores for energy. Many people have a genetic and biochemical push to make excess insulin. When insulin levels go up, the glucose in our blood drops as it is driven into our tissues and the excess insulin signals our brain to eat more food. Insulin drives us to eat more carbohydrates to replenish the blood sugar. This cycle spins out of control as more sugar in our diet increases insulin levels and more insulin drives us to add more sugar to the diet. Around and around this process goes and because we are eating excess calories at the same time, the sugar that we cannot burn is converted into fat. I measure fasting insulin in my obese patients. It is rare to find normal insulin levels. Most of the levels are 2, 3, 4 and even 5 times higher than they should be. Normal fasting insulin levels should be under 10. Fasting insulin levels under 5 are even better. I routinely see fasting insulin levels in the 25 to 50 range in obese patients. Until the diet is corrected and the overeating and excess carbohydrate intake is controlled, these elevated insulin levels will drive appetite and fat production. I will teach you how to reduce insulin levels through proper food selection and eating patterns. Some overweight patients require supplements or medication initially to assist in breaking this abnormal hormone signaling pattern.

Other hormones are at play in the weight gain phenomenon. Ghrelin and leptin play big roles. Ghrelin is a hormone produced in the stomach that signals the brain to eat. When the stomach is empty, Ghrelin is produced at higher levels. When the stomach is full, Ghrelin production is suppressed. It's understandable that some people can have abnormal production levels of this hormone making them hungry more often. Leptin is a hormone produced by our fat cells and it is designed to signal to our brain that we have had enough to eat. There are people that have low leptin levels that will make them eat more than they need to since their brain doesn't receive the proper signal that they have had enough to eat.

There are still other hormones that when not balanced can cause obesity. Thyroid hormone levels that are low will slow our body's metabolic rate and lower our body temperature. Patients with low thyroid function will gain fat quickly and retain fluids more readily. Evaluation and treatment of abnormal thyroid levels is mandatory for the obese patient. Cortisol is a hormone produced in the adrenal glands. This is our stress hormone. When the body is under intense stress from either physical or emotional causes, the adrenal glands ramp up production of cortisol. This hormone is designed to protect the body during these times of stress, but one of its effects is to stimulate production of fat. Constant daily stress that we see so often in our modern overwhelming lives, leads to steady overproduction of cortisol and the continuous production of fat. As time goes on, scientists are discovering more and more chemical substances and molecules in the body. We are only scratching the surface of the number of brain transmitters and hormone-like substances that influence and control the systems in the body. It is likely that over time we will find hundreds, if not thousands of new biologic messenger chemicals in our brain and body that have either a positive effect on our weight or a negative effect leading to the ability for easy and rapid weight gain. Knowing that our hormones play such a significant role in weight gain will allow you to combat the problem by receiving proper treatment.

ENVIRONMENT

Our current environment is conducive to weight gain. A colleague of mine coined the term "Obesigenic", meaning causing obesity. Our environment is obesigenic. We live a more sedentary lifestyle than our forefathers and mothers. We spend many hours in front of TV screens and computer screens. It's hard to believe but many people actually watch other people fish, golf, and bowl instead of doing it themselves. We enjoy the easy chair and the couch as tools of relaxation from our stressful daily work lives. We eat convenient food or "fast food", which is calorie dense and mostly combinations of fats and carbohydrates which, as explained previously, will overstimulate the brain pleasure chemicals and create an added desire to eat more. We live stressful lives which send our hormone patterns awry leading to fat production. We skip breakfast and increase our food volume as the day goes on getting most of our calories in the evening when our body doesn't require much energy. This late day eating pattern produces excess fat. In fact, Japanese Sumo Wrestlers gain their enormous body size due to nighttime feedings. I've seen many of my patients unknowingly eat the Sumo Wrestler diet.

We drink too many calories in the form of juice, sodas, and energy drinks. Even the artificially sweetened zero calorie drinks still stimulate the brain with "sweetness" and create the same pattern of over stimulation that leads to excess carbohydrate intake. Our minds are constantly stimulated with expensive marketing to get us to eat more. The marketing focuses on the "addictive" type foods such as soft drinks, snack foods, and fast food restaurant meals. We also live in a culture where more is better. Restaurants serve large portions and fast food restaurants will gladly give you a bargain on a double or supersized meal. With all of these obesigenic environmental processes going on around us, it boggles my mind when someone asks the question, "Why are Americans getting fatter?" With large marketing firms working hard to break down our resistance to bad eating and the ability to grab a quick snack or meal on nearly every street corner in any city in the country, we must learn to fight the signals and take back control of our mind and body. We are not at the mercy of other's agendas. I don't begrudge the entrepreneurial spirit and the growing companies that promote their products to us. I do want people to know that we can resist and win the battle against our obesigenic environment. I will share the treatment plans that can lead to victory over our environment as you read on.

FOOD SCIENCE

American companies are the smartest, most innovative, hardest working, and constantly improving companies in the world. Our markets and ingenuity are admired and mimicked throughout the world. When it comes to feeding the world, the United States is the leader in agricultural and food science. The technological advances made in these areas have allowed food to be grown for the entire population of the world. If not for other factors (mostly geopolitical), everyone on the planet would be able to have a daily meal. This same science that allowed mass production of food also created food processing that made foods taste better, last longer, grow faster and have greater caloric value. This highly processed food is also the culprit in over stimulating the eating centers of our brain. When the human brain is stimulated by a high density meal packed with sugar and fat, receptors are stimulated and the result is an increase in appetite for more of this food. As a result, the addiction processes in the brain are stimulated. Maybe by chance or maybe on purpose, the food processing companies have created foods that we crave. The more we eat, the more we want. The more we want, the more we eat. The cycle continues even after we realize that our body weight is getting higher and higher and we are getting physically uncomfortable with our size. The "addiction" is present and hard to break.

Many people can control their diet and the types of food that they eat for days at a time, but then satisfy the addiction with binge eating or loading up on the high calorie foods each night or on weekends. Withdrawal from these foods does not create significant symptoms such as seizures and physical sickness, though many of my food addicted patients will experience days or even a few weeks of emotional and mild physical changes when these foods are eliminated from the diet. Food scientists can create flavors that appeal to us. Any food can be textured and colored to look appealing. Food aromas can be used to stimulate our appetite (ever walk by a cookie shop in the mall?). Over the years food scientists have worked to create a snack, drink, or munchie to satisfy everyone. It's only been in the last decade that many people are becoming aware of the dangers of highly processed foods and a mini-revolution is beginning to move toward diets higher in fiber, non-modified foods, and more natural and even organically grown foods. It will take a long time for the processed food addicts to move over to organic, non-GMO, natural foods. Already, some food processors and scientists for these food companies are seeing the trend and moving away from trans-fats, high fructose corn syrup, food additives, and high gluten foods. When the population demands healthier foods in a capitalistic society, the demand will be met. It is our responsibility to break the addiction and move toward a healthier natural diet. When a large enough segment of the population moves in the direction of healthier and more natural foods, the over-processing of foods will decrease.

SOCIETY

As mentioned above, we as a society can control the type of food that we eat. Large corporations live and die by how they satisfy the masses. Many people blame McDonald's, Coca-Cola, and the other giant food companies for making us fat. They are only giving us what we are asking for. When America cried out that McDonald's was to blame for obesity, they added healthy foods to their menu. Not many people choose the healthy foods on their menu, but they are there. The responsibility lies within each of us. There is no one to blame for obesity. There are many factors involved as described above for the cause of obesity, but ultimately we are responsible to ourselves to break these bad habits and choose better quality and quantities of food. I have never accidently eaten anything in my life. Every bite was on purpose. I have never had anyone make me eat something, not counting the first year or so of my life. However, even then if I was full or didn't like the food, I would spit it out and turn my head away.

There is a societal component to weight gain, overeating, and food choice. Many people plan their days, weekends, social outings, and vacations around the meals and food they intend to eat. It is a social phenomenon to break bread with those we enjoy spending time with. Holidays have food associations with them. There are the Fourth of July cookouts, the Thanksgiving turkey and pumpkin pie. Christmas has so many foods and desserts associated with it that I can't begin to list them. Every religion has its feasts. Every country has its holidays and festivals. Food and eating are social events and eating with friends, family, and like-minded individuals is fun. Patients on reduced calorie programs will often end their program when one of these social events occurs. They don't plan to end their healthy eating plan, but the meaning placed on eating with family or friends and the meaning placed on the foods associated with holidays, festivals, and special events is strong and will overshadow our desire to have a leaner, fitter body. The psychological implications of not socializing properly during these occasions alters the meaning of the event. We eat and overeat because it's the socially accepted thing to do. If we don't comply with this social mandate, then we will feel left out, alone, and not a part of the fun. Social eating has a very strong pull on us. Many patients of mine just give up around these special times because they know the mental battle they must go through will put a damper on the occasion. It becomes easier to comply with the social norm than to rock the boat and have everyone around us wondering "what's wrong with us".

To overcome this pattern of overeating takes planning and an alternate workable blueprint on how we can maintain our lower calorie intake and still enjoy the social event while not being too conspicuous at the moment. These things are possible and when accomplished will give you a deep sense of achievement and self-control. Over time repeating this improved eating behavior will allow for the development of personal power. When this is achieved, you can approach social events, holidays, and any special occasion with confidence and control knowing that you can maintain your weight and be in charge of your future.

GOVERNMENT

I am not going to blame the government for obesity in America. I will say that when government tries to solve a problem, the fallout in the form of new problems is inevitable. Deciding that the development of a national food guide was a good idea has led to the overeating of carbohydrates in our diet. Being in charge of school lunch and eating programs, while trying to control costs, has led to poor school nutrition and the overeating of carbohydrates. Our government is now trying to fix the problem with mandated nutritional standards, but the majority of students are just saying no to mass produced poor tasting "healthy foods". When parents, teachers, and local private companies come together, as is happening in about 10% of our government run schools, good tasting healthy foods can be served to our children.

My point here is that we cannot depend or even let the massive government machine decide how we should eat and what we should eat. They've proven too big and bureaucratic to handle something as important as the health of our youth. Just as we need to truly understand how we have become fatter ourselves and the nation has become fatter, we must understand that only we can correct this problem one child and one school at a time with involvement from parents and school staff that join together with chefs, cooks, and expert nutritionists to develop local comprehensive eating programs. Even governmental control of agriculture has a deleterious effect on which foods are produced and how they are produced. For obesity to be solved in this nation, taking responsibility for the eating patterns and food choices for our own families is needed. Realizing that obesity is due to many factors and is not just caused by laziness and gluttony is going to be a requirement of our leadership in government, medicine, and education.

RESISTANCE

All of these factors play a role in the obesity epidemic that we are currently facing. They can be controlled by each of us on a personal level. But even if we understand how these factors influence eating behavior and have contributed to excess weight gain, we must also realize that overeating and poor food choices are primarily a battle in the mind. Genetics, biochemistry, food science, addiction, social patterns, and the meaning we place on food are all potent contributors to obesity, but a factor that affects all of us with regard to how we control our eating is called *Resistance*. Much of this section comes from my study of the amazingly thought provoking material of Steven Pressfield. He is an author with very strong ideas on why we as humans routinely don't accomplish the things we say we want to accomplish. I credit him with the material I am presenting here and I only hope that my ability to explain it to my readers meets with his approval. He writes about *Resistance* and overcoming it as "The" method to achieve our life's work and purpose.

As I studied his books, it became very clear to me that *Resistance* is an actual thing that gets in the way of the accomplishment of anything we want in our lives. *Resistance* is the powerful antagonist to our getting things done. For those committed to losing weight, their goals and desires are right out in front of them and on their mind every day. For others, the deep desire to reach the optimal goal weight is hidden under layers of years of frustration, self-doubt, previous weight loss failures, and pain. In terms of getting leaner, fitter, and healthier, *Resistance* exerts tremendous negative power on us. Every person who enters my weight loss and medical practice office who says they want to lose weight and become healthier, has met *Resistance* and has repeatedly come up short. I have met *Resistance* in almost every area of my own life. *Resistance* will never be permanently vanquished, but can be fought and overcome on a daily basis. We can eventually strengthen our ability to beat *Resistance*, but it is a daily fight.

Resistance occurs once we say we are committed to a task such as losing 20 pounds. At the moment we declare this to ourselves, *Resistance* rises up against us. It comes in the form of procrastination. "I will start my diet on Monday". "I will exercise tomorrow". "Just one more cookie". "Just one small piece can't hurt anything". These are the sayings that *Resistance* uses to lead us off the path that we thought we'd set for ourselves. *Resistance* comes in the form of distractions. "Work is overwhelming and I only have time to eat on the run". "My kids play sports every night and there's no time to fix a proper meal". "I'm so busy that I don't have time for breakfast". "It's our vacation and I can't be expected to stay on a diet now". All of the things that come to mind to keep us off purpose are Resistance. To fight *Resistance* requires planning, scheduling, commitment, and dedication to the task. This fight has to be undertaken on a daily basis. From the time when our eyes open in the morning until they close at night, we must be on guard against *Resistance*. Realizing that this negative force is present in us and is our enemy, we must confront it head on every day.

Acknowledging *Resistance* and understanding how it appears to us is the first step in winning the battle. *Resistance* can only be overcome by doing the work we set out to do. When we think we are in too much of a hurry to eat breakfast each day, we must plan to get up 15 minutes early and require ourselves to eat breakfast anyway, no matter what. When we feel overwhelmed at work and think that we can't take a proper break for lunch, we must plan in advance and take the lunch no matter what. When we feel that our lives are consumed by our children's afterschool and weekend activities, we must stop the whirlwind and take the time to eat a reasonable meal. Most importantly, we need to demonstrate to our children that just because life is busy, doesn't mean that we have to get our meals from a drive-thru window. Taking control of each of these situations, will beat down *Resistance* and allow for greater control of your life. Once the victories start, it is easier to become the master of *Resistance. Resistance* will never go away. It can be controlled.

How do we control *Resistance?* We must become professionals at our job. Our job is to become a lean, strong, fit, person. In using the term "professional", Pressfield is not talking about doctors and lawyers. He is speaking about professional as an ideal and a way of life. It is our job to become a professional at weight loss and weight maintenance. To overcome the obesity issue that controls our life, we must perform every day as a professional. I know that you now think I'm crazy, but it's true, becoming a professional at the thing you say you want most is the best way to actually achieve it.

Have you ever tried to learn a foreign language or play a musical instrument? If you have mastered a language or can impress someone by playing a musical instrument, then you treated the endeavor using this professional ideal. Professionals in any area do the work required even when they don't want to do the work. Think of a professional athlete or an Olympic athlete. Do you think they wanted to get up at 5am every day and practice for hours with no foreseeable reward? Do you think they enjoyed every moment of those arduous practices and training sessions? Do you believe that they were born with the talent they had and would have become a superstar anyway? The answer is that they did not enjoy the long, hard training sessions. They didn't want to always do the necessary activities to get better at their craft. They didn't even know if the hard work and effort would pay off for them in the form of a spot on the team or a chance at playing the game. They did it all because they were professionals in their attitude and behavior.

Do any of us really want to eat on plan every day? Do we want to control our eating at social events and special occasions? Do we want to exercise before or after a long day at work? The answer to these and other closely related questions is—no. We want to be thin and vibrant without having to do the work. I would love to have a magic wand to wave over myself and my patients and instantly be at our perfect weight, full of vibrancy and health. That's the thinking of a child and not of a professional. That's the talk of an amateur or a dabbler. Going on a strict dietary regimen for 2 months so that we'll look better on Spring Break is for amateurs. I'm not saying this isn't a worthy goal, but I am saying that it is short sighted and destined to end up with the same pounds lost sticking back to our bodies rapidly after the vacation ends. A professional at weight loss might set the same goal, but this would only be a sub goal in the life-long effort to keep their weight at a desired level.

Becoming a professional at health and weight management means scheduling time with your doctor or health provider to learn what is truly necessary for getting thinner for life. A professional at this endeavor would immerse themselves in the study of health and live each day within their chosen parameters. A professional will have setbacks and failures, but will immediately restart the program. Throughout this book, I will return to this philosophy of becoming a pro at losing weight and maintaining it for life. As a true weight maintenance professional, you will be able to live the remainder of your long life at your healthy desired weight. Are you ready to become a professional at losing the excess fat and a professional at maintaining a lean and healthy body? Let's work together to overcome *Resistance* and focus on our own ability to take control of our lives and beat the fat genes, the fat biochemistry, the fat creating social norms, and all of the other factors that combine to create obesity. You can win this battle and live lean, live long, and live the life you desire.

CHAPTER 5
SOLVING THE PROBLEM—BEATING THE FAT GENES

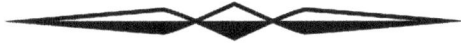

Now you know why you have struggled to lose weight and keep it off over the years. You have blamed yourself and thought that something was wrong with you. You have felt like your body was different than other people's bodies and that you were destined to stay fat. You've felt persecuted that other people thought you were lazy and an overeater because you just didn't care about yourself. You now know that your body was made to make and store fat as a protective mechanism. You know that your particular genetic makeup has made it easy to gain weight and hard to lose weight. Your hormonal and biochemical processes are geared toward appetite stimulation and cravings for sugar based foods. You've followed the guidance and recommendations of the food guide pyramid that has advised you to make the foundation of your diet a large number of carbohydrate laden and grain-based foods. You're a very busy person who takes advantage of the conveniences of modern life such as fast food restaurants and processed foods. You've become addicted to high sugar, calorie dense foods that make it hard to make significant changes in your diet. High stress in your life and the stress about carrying too much weight have perpetuated the problem by altering your sleep patterns and driving you to eat unhealthy food choices. You met *Resistance* whenever you've tried to lose weight and today, *Resistance* is winning.

Great News! You can turn all of this around. You can beat the fat genes and biochemistry. You can beat societal pressure. You can beat the addiction to sugar, fat, and processed foods. You can beat every enemy of thin. You can master *Resistance*. You can become a professional at weight loss and maintain a leaner, healthier body. Your time is now. Stop blaming yourself and commit today to taking full responsibility for becoming thin. Is this easy? No. Is this simple? Somewhat. Is this work? Yes. I know that you're not afraid of work and that you are willing to do the things that are necessary to move toward your goal weight. Stop looking for the quick fix, but realize that when doing all of the right things, your body will melt the fat off much faster than you thought. When following the correct eating and exercise patterns and dealing with the underlying disorders in the body, most obese patients will lose around 15 pounds per month. I know, you've been told to lose weight slowly so it won't come back. That's just not true. The body will drop the excess fat rapidly when put in the proper environment. My job in the remainder of this book is to help put you in the proper environment to lose the fat and keep it off. Change is not easy and most of us resist it initially. Over time and with a map to success along with accountability, you will reach your target weight and be able to live the active, fun life you've wanted to live. Now is the time. Today is day one of your new life. Let's get started.

To solve any problem, we have to think differently than we have been thinking. All of my patients in the weight loss clinic could write a book on what they know about losing weight. As I spoke about earlier, it's time to think and act like a pro when it comes to losing weight and keeping it off forever. Just knowing a lot about how to eat, how to exercise, and how to lose weight is meaningless if we don't put it into action and persist even when things aren't going our way. Being a pro means no matter what happens in our life, we remain focused on staying healthy. Taking action and being consistent are the magical ingredients to getting thin. There are specific dietary plans that work better to burn fat and specific exercise patterns that will help create lower body fat and improved muscle mass. We will go over each of these and I will give you a specific plan of attack to reach your best weight.

THE PROFESSIONAL MINDSET

Step one on Day One is to adjust your mindset. This is so much more than calories in versus calories out. No longer will we just start the diet on Monday. This is about the rest of your life and how to work toward being healthy and fit. This is about how to avoid diabetes or reverse the effects of diabetes if you currently have this diagnosis. This is about avoiding premature heart disease and the events of heart attack and stroke. This is about not being embarrassed by your body. This is about having the energy to play with your children and grandchildren. It's about enjoying your retirement and being able to travel, work in your yard, participate in your hobbies and plan new adventures no matter how old you are. Think about how you will feel wearing the clothes you've wanted to wear but couldn't fit into. Think about your slim body and others that applaud you for the accomplishment you've made and the way you look. Think about your doctor taking you off of medications that you no longer need for high blood pressure, high blood sugar, and high cholesterol. How good will you feel when the joint aches and pains go away as the pressure on the joints diminishes. You will look and feel 10 or 20 years younger in this new lean, fit, and strong body. You will have turned back the clock on aging and feel better than you have in decades. These are the things that I want you to focus on each and every day.

The diet, exercise and the accountability are the tasks that need to be done each day. Being able to perform the tasks with the mindset of a professional will lead you to the desired results. Your time of being a weight loss and dieting dabbler are over. No longer will you start a reduced calorie eating plan only to give in to temptation within the week. The professional can eat a dessert or tasty treat, but does it as part of the plan. When you encounter setbacks or reach a plateau, you will see this only as an obstacle that will make you stronger and better for having overcome it. You will learn to rejoice in your daily victories, but to stay positive throughout any adversity. You will work on your daily healthy tasks like an Olympic athlete in preparation for the single event not just to go for the gold medal but to be the best she can be at what she is doing. Just like the neurosurgeon who trains for years to hone his skills before performing meticulous brain surgery, you will be in training daily and hone your weight control skills so that over time they become ingrained in your daily behavior without you even needing to think about them.

You will understand your body and how it responds to food and activity. You will know what proper portion sizes are and how many calories your body requires. You will see your body as an incredibly made high performance machine that operates at peak capacity when the right type and quantity of fuel is provided at the right time. You will engineer your life to be just as you want it. You will be honest with yourself and stop the denial and delusions that you thought were keeping you from getting to your ideal weight. As a professional you understand that studying, self-monitoring, being accountable, and doing the things that you may not like at the moment, will lead to wonderful results in the future. You will get an attitude of "pay now, play later", rather than "play now, pay later". The future will surely come and the professional prepares today for that time. Don't be like the patients I see in their 50's, 60's, 70's, and beyond that lament that they didn't take better care of themselves when they were younger and now have to deal with multiple medications, inability to get around well, and high risk of disease and death. Resolve now to take

100% responsibility for becoming the person you truly want to be. Be your absolute best. Be a professional.

Thinking that by taking a supplement or even a diet medication, the work will be done is delusional thinking. It is amateur thinking. The professional mindset for losing weight and maintaining a healthier weight can be defined. You may think that it is hard to be a professional at anything, but you are already a professional. If you work at a job, you are a professional. Pressfield says that by working for a paycheck and receiving money for that work, you are a professional. What characteristics define the professional? Pressfield believes these are the characteristics of the professional.

1. Professionals show up every day.
2. Professionals show up no matter what.
3. Professionals stay on the job all day.
4. Professionals are committed over the long haul.
5. The stakes are high and real.
6. We accept reward for our labor.
7. We do not over-identify with the job.
8. We master the technique of our job.
9. We have a sense of humor about our job.
10. We receive praise or blame in the real world.

These characteristics that apply to being a professional in our job can also be applied to being a professional at weight loss and maintenance. Let's look at the how a professional views the job of weight loss.

1. *The professional at weight loss shows up every day.* This means that every morning when you awake, you are fully engaged in getting leaner and healthier. It may

be difficult and you may be tired and you may feel like there is no hope for you, but you do it anyway.

2. *The professional weight loser shows up no matter what.* When you step on the scales and the weight goes up or doesn't drop, you still are committed to the process of eating less and exercising more.

3. *The professional weight loser stays with the task all day.* You stay with the program until your eyes close on your pillow at the end of the day. You may think of sweets and snacks and you may crave something not on the eating plan, but you work diligently through this the entire day.

4. *The professional weight loser is committed over the long haul.* This is not a one week or one month process. This is a lifetime battle that we are going to win. Through ups and downs, vacations and travel, moods and fits, winter and summer, we are going to stay the course and live life at our lean and healthy weight.

5. *The stakes are high and real.* We understand and know without doubt that our lives depend on this mission to be successful. To live an active and long life and leave this earth while on our own two feet and not in a wheelchair, scooter, or nursing home, we must do the work of getting fit and healthy and keeping our body in the best performing state that we can.

6. *We accept reward for our labor.* When we lose enough weight for others to notice, we should accept the compliment and the payoff for our hard work. When we now fit in more fashionable and

comfortable clothes, we should pat ourselves on the back and turn this feedback into greater resolve and motivation. Be a gracious victor.

7. *We do not over-identify with our weight and our weight loss endeavor.* We work on our weight daily and for the whole day. We count our calories or carbs, and record our daily data. We track our physical activity and graph our weight reduction. We feel sometimes like our entire life centers around weight loss. It does not!! We are much more than our weight and our ability to control it. We are wonderfully created and can offer as much to the world at the beginning of our weight loss journey as we can when we are living lean. Whether we lose 2 or 3 or more pounds this week, doesn't change who we really are. We are as important to this society and world as anyone else. Because we are a professional at our weight loss endeavor, we don't identify as a fat person, thin person, or dieter. We cannot be boxed into that narrow path of living.

8. *We master the technique of losing weight and keeping it off.* We study, learn, and execute the tasks of getting leaner, fitter, and healthier. We know what we must do and we do it. We don't constantly change our ways or our plan based on the latest article in a supermarket tabloid on how some Hollywood star lost 30 pounds on the latest fad cabbage, juice, and laxative diet. We know our bodies and our life's eating and exercising plan and we stick to it.

9. *We have a sense of humor about our weight loss program.* It's OK to be un-serious as you do this. Have fun. Smile and let your optimism shine through your face. When you make a mistake or do something silly or go off the rails of your plan, don't beat yourself up. Have a laugh, realize you enjoyed the candy bar, pizza, or beer and move ahead. Resolve to be more in control, but let the past go with a wink and a smile. Life is way too short to be a self-critic every day.

10. *We receive praise or blame in the real world.* As we move through life's journey of getting and staying lean and fit, we will receive praise from many and blame or criticism from others. When I've been at my goal weight, many will tell me I'm too thin, or look gaunt, or have lost too much weight. These comments are statements about themselves and not us. To criticize us for achieving our right body size, is simply stating that they are not happy with their body or life. Accept the praise and when any criticism comes, simply say to yourself . . . "What others think about me is none of my business".

Resistance which is the enemy of our success in this and any other worthy goal or endeavor, loves the mindset of the amateur and can be defeated or at least held at bay by the professional mindset you are now guided by. You can and will be a professional at getting to your ideal body weight and maintaining it, when you plan and start the work and do it every day no matter what. Live in this professional mindset and you will live lean, live long, and truly live a rewarding life.

TAKING MASSIVE ACTION

The journey of a thousand miles begins with a single step. To finish the journey will take a massive number of steps. Each step is doable and repeatable but nevertheless it takes much, much more than the single step. I've started hundreds of "diets" and finished them on the same day. Only when I decided to take Massive Action and aggressively dedicate myself to the solution did I complete the journey. It's like the rocket that's going into space. Most of the fuel is burned and energy expended just leaving the launch pad and gaining enough momentum to leave the atmosphere. Once the velocity to leave the atmosphere is achieved, no further fuel is even required to keep it in orbit. Losing weight is much like this. Most of the activity and work occurs in the first few weeks when we are converting our body from an energy plant that uses sugar as its primary fuel to one that uses fat as its primary fuel. These initial days require the most focus and action. Once we enter the enhanced fat burning stage, we can maintain this weight loss over time with less effort. The daily major activity must be continued to keep the process going. The mechanics now become routine.

When someone is going to learn to speak and understand a new language, they must take massive action. Daily study, daily practice, and daily immersion are required or the end result will be knowing a few foreign phrases and nothing more. Learning to play the piano or the guitar require this same amount of activity. Weight loss is no different. Daily study, focus and immersion into the world of healthy eating, moderate physical activity, and accountability are required to reach the target of a lean and fit body. Over the years of running a weight loss clinic and treating obesity, I have seen many patients who say they want to lose weight, but really would prefer that someone else to do it for them. Wouldn't we all. Getting to a leaner weight is work. When you understand the amount of work, effort, and consistency that is needed, you can reach the result as long as you put in the action. Massive action gets massive results. When you start on your new dietary and activity plan to move to the end result of vibrant health, you must immerse yourself in the process. Start everyday with your result in mind. Step on the scale to tell yourself you are fully committed to the project. Keep a chart or graph of your progress. Track your food, calorie, carb, or fat intake depending on how your body loses weight the best. Look at your daily progress. Pat yourself on the back when you complete your daily task. Focus all of your effort and energy on winning one day at a time.

DAY ONE THINKING

I like to think to myself in a way I call "Day One Thinking". Every day is Day One. No matter what I did yesterday, today is "Day One". Remember how you feel on the first day of anything in your life. Remember the first day of school each year? It was exciting and full of possibility. How about the first day of a new job. Anticipation and potential were again at the top of your mind. The first days of a new relationship are always promising and hopeful. One of the best "Day Ones" is the first day of a vacation. The excitement is always palpable and the sense of freedom is amazing. When we start a new dietary regimen or a new exercise program that we know is the way we should be living the rest of our life, we again are excited, hopeful, and full of energy to get the project underway. Congratulate yourself on the days you stay totally on target. For the occasional time you slip up or stray from your plan, learn from it and start Day One all over again with the same sense of promise.

Using the ideas of Massive Action and Day One Thinking, you should be able to keep an improved focus and see better results. We have to arm ourselves in a way that allows us to permanently change our behavior. Just "trying" to lose weight and get healthy will not get the job done. Trying anything is a futile effort. We do something or we do not do something. Trying is like tasting. We are never finished and never fully satisfied.

STAY ON PATH

Every day there is a new magazine article or TV story or news show about how-to lose weight. There are new supplements or products available that are the magical answer to our weight problem. Hours of TV infomercials extoll the amazing body shaping ability of the new $1000 machine. Certainly, people can use these products and devices as tools to help them get fitter and healthier. Make no mistake, however, that these tools will not do the work for us. There is no pill, prescription or device that will melt the fat away. There is no machine or device that will take pounds away. There is no easy fix. Think seriously about this for a minute. If any advertised pill, shake, bar, device, or machine consistently turned our fat bodies into lean and trim bodies, everyone on the planet would be skinny. Once something really worked to thin us out without any effort, the news of this would travel like a virus to everyone on the planet and we would all partake of the magic. You should always read the fine print which always states "results are not typical", and "when used in conjunction with a low calorie diet and exercise".

I believe that tools are helpful. I use several tools myself. I use a step counting device which syncs to my cell phone and links to a calorie counting app, so at the end of each day I have a strong picture of what I did to stay on track to maintain my healthy weight. I use portion controlled meal replacements, protein shakes and bars, and supplements that help my body operate as efficiently as possible. I have a set of scales that measures my body weight, fat, water, and muscle mass. It sends the data to my laptop and plots a graph of my progress or maintenance. Are these tools necessary? No. They are just helpful. Do you need to spend a lot of money for tools? No. Your plan can be fully executed and the results can be amazing without any fancy or high tech tools. You can use a pencil and paper to record your daily numbers. You can read labels and ask restaurants for calorie and nutritional content on the foods you are eating. You can work out at home, in the mall or in the neighborhood without ever spending a dime for a gym or special workout clothes. When the will to lose the fat and get healthy is strong enough and the plan has been formulated with the goals in mind, you will accomplish whatever you set out to accomplish. The path to fitness and a thin body is right in front of you. Just make the decision to get started . . . today!

BREAKING THE SUGAR AND PROCESSED FOOD ADDICTION

How do we break the addiction to processed and sugar based foods? A well trained bariatric physician can assist you with this process. It can be done without medical intervention, although it may be more difficult. Going from a high sugar diet to a plant based and lean protein diet is not easy, especially if you have conditioned your body and brain over the years to rely on the white carbohydrate foods. Breads, potatoes, pasta, rice, and all of the snacks and desserts derived from these grain-based foods are sugar-based foods. For many people, the more of these foods they eat, the more of these foods they want. These are not "bad" foods. We just eat way too many of them. An occasional treat and a small amount of pure pleasure eating once in a while enhances our lives. I think that going to the new restaurant to have a memorable time and meal or having a wonderful piece of birthday cake or special holiday treat makes life a bit more rewarding and enjoyable. Knowing how to control our cravings and our food intake during these festive times is important to maintaining a healthy body. Learning to love foods that are the best for our body is the ideal answer for us to stay fit and trim for the long term.

I've never been a fanatic about health foods, organic foods or non-GMO foods, but I see the value in moving our diets in that direction. It is time to become a fanatic about breaking the sugar and processed food addiction. When an alcoholic or drug addicted patient comes into my office, I don't judge them for how they developed the unhealthy and bad habit. I feel that it is my job to help them break the addiction. The same holds true for my food addicted patients. It's important to understand their past eating habits and behavior so that I can find out specifically why they have gained so much weight. That will allow me to design a plan of attack for them to be able to conquer their addiction and to reverse the fat accumulation. To first stop the addiction, we must stop the intake of addicting foods. No alcoholic ever stopped alcohol addiction by drinking just a bit less. No one ever stops cigarettes by just cutting back. A cocaine addict can't just partake on Friday and Saturday night. The addicting substance must be eliminated from the body and no further intake can occur. Unfortunately, with food there is not such an easy answer. I'm not saying that getting off the other addicting substances is easy. In fact, the vast majority of the time it can only be done with medical supervision in a rehab center. What I am saying is that we can totally eliminate, nicotine, alcohol, cocaine, and other addictive substances from use and still survive. We cannot stop eating. No matter what we do, we will encounter and eat foods that have carbohydrates, and sugars in them.

To break the sugar addiction, however, a period of time away from the sweet stuff is necessary. I have my sugar addicted patients go through a short 3 day induction period where they avoid all sugar and grain based foods. After this short phase, their body is burning a higher percentage of fat and keeping the carbohydrates below 100 grams a day can keep the addictive behavior at bay. I don't allow refined sugar products to be eaten throughout the fat loss phase, since this can stimulate the addictive behavior. During the fat loss phase of a program, my coaches and I work to have the patient develop new long term behavior patterns and to teach them how to have a sugary treat or snack in the future without moving back into the addictive behavior pattern. Once significant body fat is lost and the feeling of euphoria about their body, health, and progress is present, new patterns can be more easily anchored to our mind. This excited state that comes from winning the battle over obesity is the exact state of mind needed to ingrain new eating behavior. Linking this new behavior to the powerful feeling of success and to the enjoyment of eating healthier foods can create new programs in the brain that make it easier for us live a leaner life.

It's important to learn that eating sweets when we're down, or when we're bored, or celebrating, or with any powerful emotion will move us back toward the addictive behavior. Many of my patients regain weight when they are stressed. Using sugar as a soothing drug during times of stress creates a powerful addictive link in our brains. We must find other methods of dealing with stress rather than opening a carton of ice cream. I use medications to help stress eaters. Helping them to deal with these emotions through the use of appropriate medication and counseling can be very effective in blocking the addiction.

Medications that stabilize the levels of serotonin and norepinephrine can be helpful in decreasing the urge to eat when stress occurs. I prescribe SSRI's such as sertraline, escitalopram, and fluoxetine for stress eating. People who tolerate these non-addicting anti-anxiety medications feel calm and have a lower response to stress in their lives. They are able to deal with the stressors better and can control the cravings for snack food which they have routinely used as a coping mechanism for stress. Sugars and sweets, in particular, have an effect in the brain to elicit dopamine release which temporarily makes us feel better. By treating patients with an anti-anxiety medication, the body and mind's response to stress is decreased and the urge to use food as a treatment for the stressful situation is diminished. For severe eating disorders, adding psychological counseling is important for altering eating behavior. Food addiction is much different from addiction to nicotine, narcotics, and amphetamines, since the withdrawal response is much, much less. People don't seize, shake, vomit, or die from withdrawal from sugar. Many of my patients do feel different and describe irritability, fatigue, stomach queasiness, and other mild symptoms associated with stopping processed foods and high sugar-based foods.

When I have patients stop sweets and dramatically reduce or stop the white carbohydrate foods such as potatoes, breads, rice, and pasta, I make sure they are getting adequate protein and a source of healthier carbohydrates from colorful vegetables. To stop the cravings for sugars and processed foods, I often need to give the patient appetite suppression therapy. Appetite suppressants can be prescription medications such as phentermine and diethylpropion or natural substances that mimic the stimulant behavior of the prescription drugs. Certain foods also have appetite suppression effects and their use can be encouraged as a regular part of the new dietary regimen. The goal is to break the addictive pattern. Treating the patient to overcome the physiological and psychological patterns can allow them to adhere to a new and healthier lower calorie diet. Just as with all addictions, if the patient returns to the original eating patterns of consuming simple sugars, high carbs, and processed foods, the addiction will return and the weight and fat problem will rapidly recur.

BEATING RESISTANCE

I have spoken about *Resistance* as an enemy of thin. Without being too redundant, I want to cover *Resistance* in more detail. The way to beat *Resistance* is to take action. Our mind will come up with a million excuses why we don't have to lose the weight. It will find every distraction and excuse available to block us from taking consistent effective action. Although we logically understand the reason why we want to lose the excess fat and get leaner, the evil forces mount against us and take us off track or worse yet, prevent us from even getting started. This is a battle and we must learn how to overcome the enemy. Remember, the enemy known as *Resistance* comes from within us. Ultimately, we can win this fight one day at a time by doing the work even when we don't feel like doing it. We perform the task of lower calorie, healthier eating even when all of the signals around us are screaming to eat the cookies, cakes, and candy. When we overcome each small battle, we build strength to continue on our mission. Will *Resistance* ever completely leave us alone? No. It's part of our nature. It's part of our socialization. It's part of who we are. Beating *Resistance* means we have to change our behavior. We may have to change who we associate with.

If all of our friends or family are overweight and don't seem to want to fight the battle, we must spend less time around them. Love them for where they're at, but don't hang around them. When you start to win the battle against *Resistance*, new friends and fellow warriors will appear. They will be a new source of strength and encouragement and will help you through their example of eating better and being more active. Actively search out others who are getting the results that you are looking to achieve. Over time, we tend to adapt the qualities of the 5 people we spend the most time with. Find 5 people that are consistently eating and exercising in a way to keep them at a healthy lean weight. Better yet, find 5 people who have struggled with weight loss and have beaten the enemy and are consistently overcoming *Resistance* and taking massive action against the causes of fat accumulation and become a part of their circle.

Most of us have to live every day in a way to overcome the fat genes, fat chemistry, fat social issues, and the *Resistance* that holds us back. We welcome others who are working or struggling with the same problems. Find positive and encouraging people and put them around you. They will hold you accountable and be a great resource to overcome the *Resistance* that has beaten you down in the past. *Resistance* can be created by interactions within your own family. This is more difficult to beat. Other people's *Resistance* will affect your path. When you are committed to eating a lean meal and everyone in the family wants a large triple topping pizza, resistance is raising its ugly head. Our family has a way of making us feel more guilty and causing us to let down our guard than others. Since they are the most important people in our lives, we give in to this group *Resistance* more readily in order to appease them. Weight loss is not about appeasement. Our family and close friends don't fight us on purpose, though it often seems that they do. They care the most for us and don't want to see us fail or be disappointed. By subconsciously sabotaging our weight loss effort, they are attempting to save us from our pain of dieting and failing in our weight loss attempt. Their opposition to helping us lose weight is more about them than it is about us.

In these situations, you must stand firm and take action to live the life you say you are committed to living. Let the pizza go and eat what you had planned on eating. Ignore any chiding or comments since they are only the problem or issue of the commenter. Be strong and realize that this is an opportunity to beat *Resistance* one more time. Stay the course, take the appropriate action, and then relish the feeling of accomplishment. Don't celebrate the victory for long though, as *Resistance* will occur just around the next corner. Excusitis and "rational lies" will pop up with each meal and at every event. These are the weapons of *Resistance*. At the moment of truth, the choice is whether to eat a portion controlled meal or to throw caution to the wind. The right decision must be made and immediately acted on to overcome *Resistance*. You can do this. Is it easy? No. Is it doable? Yes! Think about all of the times that Resistance has set you back on your path to Thin. Think of how badly you felt when you gave in to temptation. Resolve to beat *Resistance* and to fight the battle one step at a time. By fighting it every time, you will win and live a life of health, fitness, and energy. You will look great, feel great, and be great as you were intended to be. You will do the things you want to do, and live the life you want to live.

CHAPTER 6
VICTORY OVER FAT—YOUR JOURNEY TO FOREVER THIN

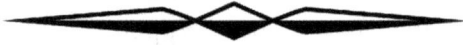

Let's talk about you. If you're reading this book, you want to know how it can help you get to your goal weight. How can you get to this? What can you do to live forever thin? The information and the ideas above have now brought you to the point of taking personal action. Living a life of personal responsibility no matter what factors and enemies have created an overweight body is the answer. If you have made it to this point and are not willing to make the effort to effect change and consistency in your life, then you must accept where you are at and live life the best you can. I believe that you would have never picked up this book or one of the many other weight loss books, articles, magazines, or programs that you have read or participated in if you didn't really want to live life to the fullest in a healthy, lean body.

I know this because I have also read all of the books, been to every seminar, signed up for every weight loss program, and had one failed experience after another. I finally came to the understanding that I had multiple factors in my life that made it easy to gain weight and hard to lose weight. It was not just about going on a diet and trying to get more exercise. Though these are a part of the thinning process, I realized that there was no easy answer. I understood that even after I reached an ideal weight, I was not cured of this disease. Only then did I accept that I would have to work at this every day. I knew that the only way to succeed was making the habits of health and beating the enemies of lean a focus of my life. I knew that I could overcome any obstacle. I was in sole control of my destiny and how I treated my body. No one ever made me eat something and I never accidently ate anything. Whether I exercised on the treadmill or got some other form of physical activity each day was under my control. I knew that I had daily demons to battle, but I was willing to go to war to maintain a healthy and fully functioning body. You can do it too!

It is now time to prepare you for the battle against excess fat and the poor health that will most certainly come from obesity. Let's first focus on a vision. A vision is what we see. In our mind, we can have a vision of our future. It's important to know where we are going if we ever plan to get there. Just saying I need to lose a few pounds will never get us anywhere. It's like saying, "I want more money". Just saying it will never make it happen. It will only come with a strong vision of the end result, a plan to get there and aggressive action to accomplish the mission. We must convince our mind that this is one of the most important things in our life. Don't downplay this fact. Without health and vitality, nothing else will matter. You will even become unable to enjoy your family and those you hold most dear.

Without health, you will become unable to leave the house and you may lose the ability to be mobile. Look around the next time you're in a large store and see how many people are using a motorized device to get around due to disability from obesity. This is not for you. When our health breaks down, it becomes the number one thing on our mind. Getting healthy and fit and staying lean and strong will add many active and exciting years to your life and to the relationships with those you love. You must be ready to reduce your body fat and total weight to healthy levels. I will use both my personal and professional experience to move you forward on your journey to becoming lean forever. I will be your partner in the process and you will succeed at achieving a lean, fit, strong, and energetic body. Feel free to LEAN on me.

TAKING ACTION—STEPS TO SUCCESS

It is the time to lose the fat and keep it off forever. There are certain things that must be done to turn your body from a fat storing machine into a fat burning machine. All these things can be done. Having a definite plan of action will make it much easier to follow along the path to thin. The plan encompasses diagnosis of the correct cause of your obesity, its proper treatment, and the evaluation of the response to treatment and modification until proper results are obtained. I will break down the step by step approach in each of these categories. When you follow the plan and are persistent, you will be able to make a major positive change in your health and life. You will become Lean.

DIAGNOSIS

As I outlined in previous chapters, it is imperative to understand why you gain weight easily and why it is difficult for you to lose weight. It is so much more than eating less and exercising more for most obese individuals. To obtain the proper diagnosis, it is necessary to find a doctor or practitioner with experience in obesity and weight management. An evaluation of the problem including a family history of obesity, diabetes, or lipid problems is required. Knowing when your weight problem began is key. Discussing what type of foods you prefer and are drawn to eat along with your eating schedule is also very important. Reviewing your activity level and any barriers to exercise is required. After a review of your personal history and family history and eating patterns, an examination of the body composition and brief physical exam will assist with recommendations for a treatment plan. Specific blood tests are also needed to measure current metabolic processes and hormonal levels in the body. I also get an EKG to assess cardiac status in case I need to use any medications in my treatment plan. Our clinic gets a metabolic assessment which tells us Resting Energy Expenditure (the number of calories used by our body to maintain vital functions) and Exercise Energy Expenditure for varying levels of exercise. The collection of this data allows us to get a better understanding of each person's weight issues. With this knowledge, a specific program can be established that is best for each patient. All lower calorie diets will work if someone stays on them long enough. The problem occurs when the diet plan is complete and a person reaches their goal weight. This because there is a tendency to regain the weight because the underlying problem has not been addressed.

Commercial programs, which have great eating and exercise plans along with some counseling, will work for short term weight loss. Unless the specific cause of the obesity disorder is corrected or controlled, the weight will return fairly rapidly. Even patients who have bariatric surgical procedures have a high rate of return of weight and fat within a few years of the procedure if the underlying hormonal, biochemical, psychological and hereditary factors are not evaluated and treated. A total of 90–95% of all people will gain most, if not all, of their weight back within a 5 year period. The percent is less with bariatric surgery such as Roux en Y or gastric sleeve procedures, but the average weight loss at 5 years is about on a par with any supervised long term medical weight loss program.

To make the diagnosis simpler, I have listed in bullet point fashion the evaluation process and testing specifics. Each physician may have some varying tests that they prefer in making their diagnosis of the cause of obesity in each of their patients.

DIAGNOSTIC EVALUATION OF OBESITY

1. Patient and family history of any disease, illness, and specifics about their obesity problem

2. Current medication list

3. Physical Examination

4. EKG, if medications are contemplated

5. Blood tests including: CBC, chemistry assessment, thyroid panel, glucose evaluation (A1c, insulin level, glucose), lipid study and hormonal evaluation of estrogens and androgens in appropriate patients

6. Body composition and metabolic rate analysis

7. Discussion and evaluation of stress, depression, anxiety and substance use

8. Psychological eating assessment

Once these evaluations and studies have been performed and the data returned, a specific treatment protocol can be offered. I have found that when patients have an understanding of "why" they have gained so much weight and "why" they have trouble controlling their calorie intake along with what drives them to eat certain foods, the results of the treatment are much faster and better than just going on the next diet and exercise program.

By treating obesity as a disease, which it is, I advise my patients that the treatment plan will not cure their obesity. The disorder is with them for their entire life. That statement can be devastating for some patients. It is because they are looking for a "cure" and a once and for all fix so they can be thin for the rest of their lives. They can be thin the rest of their lives but they also must treat the disease the rest of their lives. Treating obesity is no different than treating hypertension or asthma. These disorders don't go away. They can improve or worsen over time depending on lifestyle, exposure to external factors, and intensity of treatment, but they are always with the patient. When the hypertension or asthma are under control, we say they are in remission.

When an overweight patient reaches their goal weight and holds that weight, I tell them that they are in remission. When an asthma patient has an episode of wheezing and breathing problems, they are having an "asthma attack". When one of my obesity patients in remission gains more than 5% of their body weight back, I tell them they are having a "Fat Attack" and must return for immediate treatment of the disorder. The underlying disorders that caused the original weight gain have broken through and the eating and activity patterns can return to the obesogenic pattern. The diagnosis is critical to proper long term care of each patient and for each patient to understand their body's own tendency to gain weight. It is very important to look for proper evaluation and treatment of obesity and abnormal weight gain. There are many commercial programs in storefronts, as well as online and mail order programs that will assist in the weight and fat loss process. All of these programs focus on eating a calorie deficient diet which will result in weight loss.

I commend these various plans and programs. However, most of them only approach obesity as a problem to be fixed in the short term. "Come in" or "order now" and lose weight this week. "Get in shape for summer". These programs, for the most part, will work for a short period of time; but, without figuring out the underlying reasons that the person has gained weight, a cookie cutter one-plan-fits-all diet will lead to a weight loss–weight gain cycle and frustration. Our programs see those same patients who have been led to believe through marketing that this is a disorder that can be eliminated once your goal weight is achieved. We cannot treat obesity like we treat a cold. I believe that the addition of a thorough diagnostic evaluation and proper treatment of the disorder along with a commercial or medical program and regular counseling by trained weight management professionals can lead to many more people reaching and maintaining their appropriate weight. I have patients who have been on a local commercial program off and on for years and have not seen any long term progress. Once we find the underlying causes for their obesity and establish a plan to treat it, the same commercial program that they like, seems to work much better as the patients will tell and show me.

If any single program, product or diet on the market could actually permanently produce weight loss for everyone and each and every person reached their ideal weight and kept it off, then that program or product would control the market and everyone would be thin. I encourage people to choose a dietary regimen that they can enjoy, tolerate, and stay on for a long time whether that's my eating plans or someone else's. However, I do require an initial evaluation and diagnosis and add the appropriate treatment to their dietary regimen. Diet is only one part of the weight loss solution. Anyone that is obese and thinks that dieting alone will lead to lifetime of lean living will live a very frustrating and persistently obese life. This is no different than a person who thinks that taking an appetite suppressant is the answer to their problem without changing their diet or activity level. They are fooling themselves. Appetite suppressants play an important role but in and of themselves will not create lasting weight loss. This holds true for exercise without the other components of a solid program. A sound plan that encompasses all of the necessary treatment modalities for obesity will work on anyone and if followed for life can lead to living the remainder of your life at your ideal weight.

TREATMENT OF OBESITY

1. Establish patient acceptance of and commitment to treating the disease of obesity

2. Definitive diagnosis of the cause of the disorder—hormonal, addiction, psychological, genetic, co-morbid process, or a combination

3. Designed reduced calorie eating plan based on diagnostic evaluation

4. Prescribed activity program based on patients ability, size, and experience

5. Daily self-monitoring program

6. Appetite suppression through food selection, supplements, or medication

7. Medication therapy to combat specific disorders leading to the obesity such as hormonal imbalances, insulin resistance, stress eating and sleep disorders

8. Counseling and treatment for psychological problems that promote the obesity

9. Education regarding the body's expected response to weight loss

10. Goals that are realistic, but require a stretch

11. Regular accountability and long term follow up with provider and coaches

12. Easy and empathetic access to and re-entry into the program for relapse at its earliest occurrence.

13. Lifetime follow up as with any chronic disease.

Many of the commercial and online programs do have several of these treatment requirements, but without medical evaluation and additional treatment, long term remission is extremely difficult to achieve. Many estimates dealing with how many patients lose substantial weight (greater than 30 pounds) and keep it off for greater than 5 years reveal dismal numbers. The number is right around 5%. That means that 95% of the people that change their diets, exercise, join programs, spend hundreds or thousands of dollars, and commit to changes will end up gaining the lost weight back within 5 years and often earlier. This tells me that the current management of obesity is poor. Both the understanding of long term weight loss by the patient and the focus of most programs are short term and result in only partially treating the disorder. Current therapy focuses on reducing calories and increasing activity until a goal weight is achieved. Patients and programs don't see the patient again until the weight has returned. This would be like treating diabetes until the blood sugars are normal and then stopping all treatment. When individuals understand that their obesity condition and weight gain tendency is a lifetime disorder, they are much more likely to make lifetime changes and to accept lifetime treatment and accountability. It is our responsibility to educate patients and to let them know that obesity is a lifetime disorder and not just a cosmetic issue to be "fixed" in a short time. Fat loss can be rapid, but the disease must be managed over the long-term. This is why many patients want bariatric surgery so that they can "fix" the problem. Surgery doesn't cure the disease and post-surgical treatment is mandatory to prevent the re-gaining of weight.

An ongoing study of people who have lost over 30 pounds and have kept it off for at least one year, provides an excellent insight into weight loss. This study, called the National Weight Control Registry, has over 10,000 individuals enrolled. Members complete annual questionnaires about their current weight, diet and exercise habits, and the behavioral strategies that they use to maintain their lower weight. The habits that they perform regularly are markedly consistent within the group. It is important to remember that these individuals have gone through the weight loss phase and are now in the remission or weight maintenance phase. Many of the same principles apply to both phases. A condensed version of many of the study's statistics revealing methods for weight loss and maintaining a lower, healthier weight are presented below. This is what successful weight losers and low-weight maintainers do.

SEVEN HABITS OF LONG TERM WEIGHT LOSS MAINTENANCE

1. Eat breakfast daily. I advise eating within 1 hour of awakening.

2. Weigh weekly. I prefer a daily weigh-in.

3. Keep TV time to under 10 hours per week. This includes non-job computer screen time.

4. Exercise daily. I advise working out up to 1 hour daily.

5. Walking was the most common physical activity for these weight losers.

6. Most of the individuals had assistance from a formal program.

7. Food intake modification was the number one common habit.

These findings should not be a surprise for anyone. The difficulty in any weight loss effort is being able to stay on track during the entire weight loss phase of the program. This can require blocking hormonal and biochemical signaling until the body can readjust its chemistry and eliminate the overriding signals that have been coming from the large amount of stored fat in the body. I am not saying that weight maintenance is easy, but there is a specific lifestyle regimen that will assist in keeping you lean. Getting to lean and staying there is the main focus of this book.

Accepting the disease of obesity and committing to its treatment is the first step. I have many patients who come to me and expect me to make them lose weight. I inform them that this is a partnership. Unless they are ready to immerse themselves in the process and program of fat loss, I will be unable to assist them in any meaningful way. My talk with them focuses on why they came to me for a weight loss solution. Most will tell me that it's because they've been on every program and the weight just keeps coming back. They believe that as a physician I have a magic pill to make them lose weight. I certainly have medications and techniques to assist them, but without full commitment, they are going to fail. Once I have full buy-in to the complexity of the disorder and the need to focus on this as one would focus on a career, the raising of a child, or any major undertaking in life, we will partner to move through the weight loss phase as rapidly and as safely as possible.

This raises the age old question of "should I lose weight slowly or rapidly"? I believe the answer is . . . it doesn't matter. As long as you are not becoming dehydrated or entering starvation, fast weight loss in a monitored situation is not unhealthy. Losing 3 or 4 pounds in a week is considered fast weight loss. Losing < 1 to 2 pounds per week is considered slow. In the National Weight Control Registry study, it was found that there was a very wide range of length of time for the weight loss to have occurred. In this study, weight loss of 30 to 300 pounds took between 1 year and 66 years. This doesn't tell us much, but a study at the University of Florida concluded that quick weight loss was a better way to lose weight than slow weight loss. In this study, the fast losers lost 1.5 pounds more per week than the slow losers. Those who lost weight fast were 5 times more likely to lose at least 10% of their body weight. Fast losers were more likely to keep a food journal and did not consume as many calories as their slow loss counterparts.

Other observations in the study revealed that quick weight losers saw greater improvement in physical appearance and heightened energy levels. These positive effects tend to increase motivation and encourage people to maintain an obesity treatment regimen. There is no evidence that slow losers or fast losers are more apt to regain the lost weight or even more weight after the loss. Individuals who go on starvation diets and become dehydrated and calorie depleted will see rapid regain after ending a program. However, much of this is rehydration which can be 4–10 pounds of fluid weight. I decided to call my weight loss clinic "Fast Clinical Weight Loss" to promote that losing a controlled weight amount in a quick time along with monitoring is appropriate and very self-motivating. I sometimes think that programs admonishing clients to only lose a pound to a pound and a half a week for safety reasons are attempting to string the client out for a long time. If you have to lose 80 pounds or more and lose a pound a week, it's certainly better than never losing the weight. However, most people won't tolerate the 80 weeks that it would take. I prefer to work with people to take massive action and get the job done, while at the same time working with them on nutritional counseling, psychological treatment, and increasing exercise regimens.

My weight loss clinic utilizes three different reduced calorie dietary regimens (which I will cover in more detail in another chapter), focused medication therapy for the root cause of the resistance to weight loss, coaching, counseling, cognitive therapy, and accountability through regular visits, emails, and phone calls. Our three dietary regimens are called LEAN programs. They incorporate a higher level of protein along with a reduced amount of carbohydrate. These are not ultra-low carbohydrate diets, but carbs are reduced enough to shift the body toward utilizing fat as its primary fuel source. Our 3 LEAN programs provide 900, 1100, and 1300 calories respectively. I use portion controlled meal replacements in each of the programs along with real food meals in two of the three plans. One plan utilizes only the portion controlled meal replacements.

Medications are prescribed in our program for problems such as hormone imbalances, carbohydrate sensitivity syndromes, stress eating patterns, and appetite suppression. Being able to combat and overcome the underlying issues that drive eating and the resultant obesity, allow for the body to lose fat and to decrease the levels of inflammation and oxidation. Inflammation and oxidation are accelerated due to excess fat in the body. These processes are dangerous and become self-perpetuating leading to cardiovascular disease, diabetes, certain cancers, and many other debilitating diseases. By reducing body fat and increasing physical activity, the inflammatory substances in the body become reduced. Eating healthier foods such as vegetables, low sugar fruits, and high fiber foods also help to control inflammation and oxidation. Inflammation is a constant irritant to cells and tissues causing them to react in negative ways. Oxidation can be thought of as "rusting" of our cells and tissues.

All of my patients know that losing weight and eating better is beneficial for their health. However, they do not necessarily understand the underlying mechanisms that are going on in the body that can either damage or heal it. I try to get them to understand that negative metabolic processes that occur from a poor diet cause damage to our arteries and organs. For instance, having too much sugar in the bloodstream will damage the lining of our arteries allowing cholesterol to get underneath the artery lining and cause plaques and blockages to occur. The sugar molecules are actually crystals which tend to scratch at the lining of our arteries. Keeping blood sugar levels down decreases this artery lining injury. The treatment of obesity is much more than losing weight to look better and feel better. It's about stopping the damage that is constantly occurring to our tissues when we carry too much fat. Excess fat over time will destroy vital cells and tissues and reduce our life expectancy by decades. Getting to a lean, healthy weight and reducing sugars in the diet will correct the negative inflammatory effects that lead to vascular and organ disease. The resultant improvement in tissue and organ function and reduction in cellular injury along with the increase in healthy longevity are the bonuses of living a leaner life. Looking better and feeling better are also great things and nice motivators to keep the weight down.

Another aspect of the treatment of obesity involves psychological evaluation as a mechanism to reprogram our thinking. I'm not talking about psychiatric treatment, but treatment of cognitive patterns that develop over time and create great resistance to our weight loss efforts. As we grow up, we associate certain meanings to food. Many mothers use food as a sign of love with their children. This process is not intentional but comes out of the need to nourish and please a child. The child also feels comfort and love from the effort and the tasty meals that are prepared by the hands of the parent. Many patients tell me that one of the most difficult things to do is to go home to their mothers and not succumb to the amazing foods that are prepared just for them. In fact, the guilt associated with not consuming these home cooked delicacies is so strong that they all return with weight gain. Many special foods are designated for holidays and religious events and seasons. Not partaking in these foods disturbs the mind and creates a sense of disassociation from the event or significance of the season. Birthday foods are a required part of the annual celebration. I've never been to a birthday party without a cake, ice cream, or some other equally wonderful confection. The same holds true for weddings where hundreds or even thousands of dollars are spent on the cake. Every American holiday is associated with a particular meal, food, or eating event. The Fourth of July cookout stands out among them. Thanksgiving and the accompanying feast has been detrimental to everyone wanting to improve their body weight and fat composition.

We place meaning on our foods that become ingrained in how we think, feel, act, and, of course, eat. Food has become much more than just nutrition. It has become a social staple in our society. Going out with friends, or visiting friends or relatives revolves around a meal. Business meetings or rather business "wining and dining" are a key part of the sales and business building program. The business people in my weight loss program struggle with being able to perform on their jobs if they don't fully participate in the business events and dinners. They feel somewhat unworthy in the business arena if they are not partaking of the food and beverages while presenting their business ideas and doing their deals.

Changing how we view food and what it means to us is not easy, but it can be done. Being able to avoid food for other reasons besides nutrition is extremely difficult. Food can be a drug used for stress. Food is a friend and companion to the lonely and bored. Food can be the answer to abuse and a history of damaging relationships. Food is our trophy in victory and our bandage in defeat. Unless we can begin to understand how we use the ingestion of food as a way to attempt to soothe our mind and emotions, then getting to our lean weight will be nearly impossible. Maintaining our lean weight over time will not happen without a shift of our thought pattern.

As a prominent psychologist, Dr. John Sklare, has said "The physical act of eating always follows the mental decision to eat". I tell my patients a very similar statement by saying "I've never accidentally eaten anything, it's always been on purpose". Reviewing some of Dr. Sklare's data reveals that psychological issues that contribute to and help cause obesity are stress eating, physical discomfort from reducing calorie intake, perfectionism, inner control issues, commitment level issues, and secondary gain issues. His analysis shows that 95% of patients have problems with at least two of these issues and that 60% of obese individuals struggle with at least three of these psychological issues. The strongest of these mental resistance patterns are stress eating, physical discomfort of reducing calories, and perfectionism. Learning how to manage the space between the decision to eat and actually eating can be a major factor in losing weight and living at a leaner weight for good. Fortunately, there are cognitive changes that can be made to improve the mind and its ability to overcome these psychological issues. A specific program of cognitive therapy will create new thought patterns to deal with the ability to make better decisions when the urge to eat arises. I provide an online psychological analysis and treatment plan for our patients as part of our overall program.

The treatment of obesity, weight issues, and the resultant poor health that comes from excess body fat is different for each individual. It is critical not to expect that a single cookie cutter diet will work for everyone. Unfortunately, over time, these types of plans fail for 95% of all individuals. Taking a well thought out path to get a proper diagnosis, specific targeted treatment which includes an eating plan, activity plan, medical therapy for specific genetic and biochemical issues, and psychological analysis and therapy will result in many individuals being able to conquer there weight problems. Most of those people who follow this path will dramatically reduce fat and improve the quality of their lives. There are many doctors and programs that can provide you with this comprehensive type of care. You don't necessarily need a doctor, nutrition expert, exercise trainer, psychologist, and program coordinator. This would be cumbersome and cost prohibitive. Most trained physicians have the staff and the ability to satisfy all of these treatment modalities in a reasonable bundled program that works to overcome all of the issues and can be undertaken for a price competitive with commercial diet programs which typically offer only 1–2 of the treatment segments. Take time to research and find the right obesity treatment program. Your life depends on it and with the proper treatment plan you can live lean, live long, and live life to the fullest.

CHAPTER 7
IMMERSION AND MASSIVE ACTION

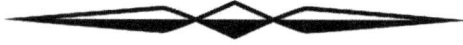

One of the most important components of losing weight and keeping it off is the degree of commitment to the effort. No matter how many times you've tried to lose weight and failed at the task, getting to your optimal weight is a worthy life goal. It will add years to your lifespan and vibrancy to those years. The process of weight loss and weight maintenance requires the highest priority that you can give it. You must immerse yourself in the task and take massive action from the beginning. As an example, how long would you give a baby time to learn to walk from the time it is able to stand? Would you give the baby a day, week, or a month? If the baby didn't walk during that time, but continued to stumble and fall, would you put an end to the child's attempts and just carry the child the rest of its life? Of course, you wouldn't. You would even say that was silly to even think such a thing. Weight loss and long term control is just like this. How long would you give yourself to make it to your goal? If you treat weight loss the same way you treated the expectation of a child to walk proficiently, you would eventually be thin for life. We give up too soon. We think that a failed attempt ends the process. We think a bad day at dieting allows us to throw in the towel. Daily immersion and massive action should become the attitude of each day during the fat loss process and for the rest of your life. This is the attitude that results in thin and healthy for life.

LONG TERM WEIGHT MAINTENANCE

It's important to discuss keeping weight off after the loss of significant fat tissue. The last thing that anyone wants is to work hard at reaching a healthy weight and then see the fat return over time. Even if you haven't yet started a weight loss treatment plan, it's important to read about what it will take to keep the weight off forever. Remember, the statistics are not in your favor. Just losing weight for the sake of hitting a short term goal will not solve the long term disorder of obesity. As previously stated, 95% of significant weight losers regain the weight and in many cases gain additional weight over their original starting weight. The disease process does not go away. The underlying biochemistry is improved with the weight and fat loss, but the genetic factors that drive the biochemistry and the environment presented to us is not in our control. If not practiced regularly, the changes we make with our thinking can drift back toward a pattern that leads to overeating. We can control and override the genetics, biochemistry, psychological, and environmental factors, but it takes daily vigilance.

The specific therapy and treatment that took the weight off must be continued on a daily basis, although modifications can occur. It doesn't take the same intensive effort to keep weight off as it does to lose the weight, but it does take regular effort in the same areas to ensure that you will live the rest of your life at a lean and healthy weight. I often tell my patients that treating a disease to get it under control and treating a disease to manage it require ongoing compliance with the treatment plan. When my patient with severely uncontrolled blood pressure presents in my office, the first goal of therapy is to lower the pressure. We then work on any correctable factors that may have contributed to the urgent situation. Once the blood pressure returns to a normal and safe range, we don't stop therapy and wish the patient well. The genetics, biochemistry, and environment that caused the high blood pressure is still there. Ongoing monitoring, control of the personal environment such as diet and exercise and treatment with medication to keep the blood pressure stabilized is necessary in most cases. This same ongoing process is needed for the treatment of obesity. Continual monitoring of the disorder, personal control of diet and exercise ongoing at home therapy for psychological and medical issues that led to the obesity is required.

There are many patients in all programs that want the initial weight loss to be the cure for the disorder. I get it. I want the same thing, but the mature and reasonable approach dictates that we treat our obesity even when the outward evidence of the disease is resolved. You may look thin, feel thin, and be energetic and healthy as a thin person should be, but the disease lies under the surface ready to rise up again at the first sign of complacency and the return to old habits. These old habits are deeply ingrained and once released will stimulate the genetics that have been overcome to create a biochemical storm that leads to overeating of the foods that stimulate our brain to want more calorie dense fat and sugar laden foods. This is not unlike a smoker who has been able to break the nicotine addiction. Subtle cravings will always come into their minds. However, as long as control is maintained and the satisfaction of the craving is not taken, then the brain chemistry that is responsible for the recurrence of the addiction will remain dormant. Once a single puff of a cigarette occurs, the full blown addiction to nicotine is immediately reactivated and the smoker is back to a pack a day habit. With sugar and highly brain stimulating foods, the analogy holds but the exact mechanisms differ. Receptors to sugar like those of nicotine have not been proposed as the addictive mechanism, but make no mistake that going back to even moderate levels of sugar, sweets, and simple carbohydrates as the mainstay of the diet will promote a chemical storm in the brain that perpetuates the excess eating behavior and cravings. It's not the single treat in moderation that does us in and leads us back toward obesity. It's the repetitive eating of a high carbohydrate, high sugar diet that leads to the production of the excess fat and the self-perpetuation of uncontrolled cravings and unhealthy eating. It's like we have two individuals inside our head. There is one telling us all of the reasons why eating the box of cookies won't hurt us and the other telling us that these cookies will only be the start of overeating and the undoing of our diligent efforts to be fit and trim. Treating this emotional and mental battle is an ongoing process. Learning new ways to deal with the choices presented to us hundreds of times a day as to what, when, why, and where to eat a meal must be a part of our thought process. Making better choices and decisions can become second nature if enough study, practice, time, and effort is put into it.

Every day, self-monitoring, eating a breakfast, getting additional exercise, planning for adequate sleep, avoiding or learning to handle stress effectively, and making eating choices based on how important it is for you to remain lean and healthy rather than a moment of pleasure are at the core of maintaining your new thinner body. If part of your weight loss plan was to combat other diseases related to the excess fat such as diabetes, hypertension, high cholesterol, arthritis, and the multitude of other co-disorders, then monitoring those disorders through regular check-ups and home self-monitoring are critically important. If you have been able to stop the negative effects of diabetes or another disease by getting to a leaner weight and reducing fat, then making sure that the parameters of the disease are stable and in a healthy range will assist you in staying committed to the long haul. Seeing your bad cholesterol levels at goal or your blood pressure in the healthy range can be a very motivating factor in making daily eating decisions.

Another method of maintaining your long term motivation is to pay close attention to the fit of the clothes you are wearing. Having comfortable, well fitting, and complimenting clothes to wear is a great feeling. If you feel that the clothes are beginning to pull or constrict, then you know that you have gone out of remission and the obesity disorder is not in control. The "Fat Attack" has occurred. Anytime one of my patients who is at their optimal weight and suddenly gains 5% of their body weight back, they are having a "Fat Attack". The attack needs to be treated aggressively and quickly to regain control of the disease and to put the disorder back into remission. Recall that just like the asthmatic having an "Asthma Attack", the obesity "Fat Attack" should be treated as an emergency. Left unchecked, the fat attack will suddenly become a 20 or 30 pound weight gain and the resultant mental and emotional anguish will feed the fire and promote even more weight gain. Guilt and withdrawal will begin and unfortunately many people who go down this path do not seek out treatment until their entire weight loss has been regained. Recognizing the signs of early weight loss and eating behavior changes can allow you to live life within 5% of your lean, healthy weight. Recognizing that this is a difficult disorder to control and that assistance is needed will save your life. No professional who is helping you will judge you for regaining some weight. They will be empathetic and excited that you understand the obesity disease process and have responded quickly and proactively to regain control of the disease and your life. When you understand this about the disease of obesity and understand the way that you should respond, then you will be able to live a lean, fit, strong, and healthy life with the body that will be under your control.

CHAPTER 8
THE LEAN PLAN—TREATING OBESITY FOR LIFE

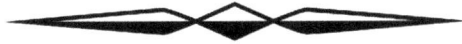

The question to answer now is . . . How do I treat my disease of Obesity? I am going to cover what I do to treat overweight and obese patients in my weight loss / weight management clinic. At <u>Fast Clinical Weight Loss</u>, my staff and I offer a customized approach to weight loss. Each person who comes in for an initial consultation has some pre-conceived ideas of how they want to lose weight and what type of program will work best for them. Unfortunately, this is a rational lie that each person tells themselves. If they truly knew t the best way for them to lose weight and keep it off, then they wouldn't even need to visit me or my office in the first place. Every person who has ever had a weight problem has attempted multiple weight loss programs, plans, and sometimes goofy and unusual processes to lose weight. Every person with a weight problem is looking for the easiest and quickest way to end their misery. What new plan, program, pill, device, or special food can I use to end the struggle with weight once and for all?

Most of my patients could write their own book on dieting, weight loss programs, and how to lose weight. What they have learned to date has not allowed them to conquer this problem. They are still living in denial that this is a lifetime disorder and that lifetime treatment and management is necessary. Many will give lip service to this, but still think that if I can help them just lose the pounds, then they will be cured and can live life the way they want, even though past experience has proven this theory wrong. I as a physician/patient want to believe this. I want to believe that one last effort to get to my goal weight will solve the problem permanently. I know it's a lie my brain wants to believe, but I also realize that my past history of losing the weight only to regain the weight is proof that I require implementation of a total plan and need to work that plan for life. Any time I deviate from the total plan, I expect to gain weight and based on my history will gain weight. I tell my patients that I am on a diet every day of my life. Am I perfect? No. I am always working at doing better.

During the initial interview, my staff discusses past successes and failures regarding weight loss and gathers information on how the patient perceives the weight loss process. Some patients are very resistant to the total treatment plan of a specific eating program, medical evaluation and therapy, psychological evaluation and treatment, and long term maintenance planning. I still treat these patients and hope that over the course of their weight loss program, I can move them toward a greater understanding of the disease and how to effectively treat it long term. The old adage applies—"If you keep doing what you're doing, you'll keep getting what you're getting". Many have come to accept this idea of total treatment and are doing well long term. Others resist and unfortunately become a patient of mine many times over and over just to lose the same weight again and again. We never give up on anyone and welcome them to stay with us and return at any time. I am never critical of a patient though I am open and honest with their efforts. My job is not to judge or be upset with a patient, but to come to an understanding of the underlying problem that the patient is having. With that knowledge, I can then attempt to partner with them to solve the issue. The components of a complete weight loss and long term weight management program include several factors.

COMPONENTS OF A COMPLETE WEIGHT MANAGEMENT PLAN

1. The Eating Plan—Changing how we eat

2. The Activity Plan—Changing how we move

3. The Mental Plan—Changing how we think

4. The Medical Plan—Improving how our body chemistry and machinery works

5. The LEAN LIFE Maintenance Plan—Staying Forever Thin

THE EATING PLAN

In our clinic, I use 3 different eating plans to give patients a reduced calorie intake. They are designed to be used individually or can be used as a 3 level step-up program of graduated calorie increase. The plans are called our "LEAN" Plans. They are all designed to provide an increase in protein intake and a decrease in carbohydrate intake. They approximate 40% protein, 40% carbohydrate and 20% fat. There is some variance in this depending upon the selections of food and snack meals on each plan. Our lowest calorie and most aggressive plan is called LEAN 7/900.

LEAN 7/900: This plan is the simplest since it provides 7 small portion-controlled meal replacements a day totaling around 900 calories with the above listed protein/carbohydrate/fat ratio. The only selections to be made are what meal replacements the patient wants. They receive a variety of different shakes, bars, puddings, oatmeal, chips, and other small meals. On this program, patients eat every 2½ hours. Hunger is not typically a problem and the usual discomfort of dieting is minimized due to the frequent meals. This plan will put the patient into increased fat burning within a short period of time and along with a therapeutic vitamin packet and specific medication when indicated, our patients lose an average of 12–15 pounds a month. Depending on the amount of weight loss needed and each patient's adherence to the plan, these results can vary. As the patient follows the 7/900 plan, we see blood sugar levels drop to low normal ranges, insulin levels drop into the normal range of below 9 and triglycerides, which are storage fats in the blood, drop dramatically. Those with elevated blood pressure and blood sugars can see dramatic improvement within a couple of weeks. I encourage our patients to drink water until their afternoon or evening urine is as clear as water. If their afternoon or evening urine is yellow or dark, they are not getting in enough water. Non-caloric beverages are allowed, but limited, as too many no-calorie sweet beverages such as diet sodas will still stimulate the brain to demand more carbohydrates and sweets. Drinking too many diet drinks will make staying on the plan more difficult since those stimulated cravings add resistance to the daily reduced calorie regimen. I like this program a lot for people who struggle with preparing foods that are lower in calories and still fit the nutritional needs similar to this 7/900 plan. There is almost no food preparation and modestly limited choices in food tend to allow people to stay on a low calorie diet plan more easily than a plan with unlimited choices. Many of our biggest fat losers have used this plan to propel them toward their optimal weight.

LEAN 51: This plan is our most popular plan and also acts as a step up plan from LEAN 7/900. This plan includes 5 portion-controlled meal replacements a day along with one meal which I call Lean and Green. Most patients take the Lean and Green meal at supper time in the early evening. On the LEAN 51 plan, the total calories consumed are between 1100 and 1200 depending upon the chosen meal replacements and the selections of the daily meal. We give specific instructions of what foods to eat for the Lean and Green meal.

Patients are again eating about every 3 hours while awake. This eliminates hunger and the desire to overeat. It is critical not to miss meals on these LEAN plans. This will lead to increased appetite and risk of overeating later in the day. The first meal of the day should be eaten within 1 hour of awakening and then every 2 ½ to 3 hours the prescribed meal replacements should be eaten. Our patients on the LEAN 51 plan will typically lose between 10–15 pounds a month, again varying based on adherence and commitment to the plan. I again treat any medical cause of weight loss resistance as needed with either natural supplements or prescription medication. The different medications I use can assist with appetite suppression, stress eating, sugar addiction, and hormonal abnormalities. Our patients are seen in follow up monthly to monitor progress and to sustain accountability. Some patients stop in more often to weigh and touch base with the coaches. We also provide a psychological eating profile on all of our LEAN plans so that our clients get a true understanding of the mental aspect of why they have struggled with weight loss and long term weight maintenance. The program is administered through a questionnaire that is statistically valid to determine the underlying psychological patterns that cause resistance to weight loss. A cognitive therapy plan which is self-administered is used to get people to improve their ability to stay on plan for the long term and to develop new behavior and thought patterns with respect to food and eating.

LEAN 3: This plan provides 3 real food meals and 3 portion-controlled meal replacements or snack meals a day. The total calorie intake on this plan varies between 1200 and 1400 calories depending on the selection of foods on the meal planner and the snack meal selection. We counsel individuals on how to choose the right foods to stay at one end of the range or the other depending on their starting weight and weight goal. This a great step up plan from the LEAN 51 plan and more closely mimics the real life eating pattern for long term weight control. The real foods focus on increasing healthy proteins in the diet and the reduction of carbohydrates, especially the white carbs such as breads, potatoes, pasta, and rice. Avoiding simple sugars is necessary to stay in the fat burning process. We have our patients self-monitor on all of the LEAN plans either with a paper journal provided in the workbook or on a computer or smartphone app. Tracking daily food intake is necessary for both weight loss and long term weight management. Anyone who says they can track this in their head is destined for a failed dietary intervention. Our coaches follow patients and assist them with any sticking points as they move through the weight loss phase of the dietary plan. Our goal is to have the patient be much more aware and mindful of both their physical and psychological eating patterns from the past and the new one's that they develop during our program. Understanding why, when, and what we eat is necessary in order to make long term healthy changes. We transition our patients to a normal eating pattern of 3 meals a day and 3 snacks a day when they have reached their optimal weight and determine their appropriate caloric need through metabolic testing. We use both electrical impedance and oxygen consumption techniques to calculate resting energy expenditure and estimated caloric usage for typical various activity amounts and patterns. This gives the patient the ability to know how much food intake they can have for a specific amount of lifestyle activity that they perform. Our goal is to have them be able to maintain a 5% variance of their goal weight. If at any time they gain back more than 5% of their optimal weight, they should see this as an emergency and return for treatment of the obesity disease, now out of remission.

THE ACTIVITY PLAN

Long term maintenance of weight and overall health depend upon getting adequate physical activity on a regular basis. When a patient starts a LEAN program and treatment in our office, we review and discuss their current level of activity. Most who are significantly overweight have very little physical activity going on in their lives. I advise them to not worry about exercise at the beginning. For most people, this is a big relief. My belief is that our weight is about what we eat, and our size or inches is about what we do. I routinely see patients who are attempting to lose weight with intensive exercise alone. They usually become very frustrated since they see no change in their weight. You cannot out train a bad eating plan. They are certainly becoming more fit. Without a change in eating patterns, they will become more fit but still fat. A change in dietary intake is necessary to lose fat and weight. I start my obese patients on a proper weight loss eating plan initially without having them worry about exercise. When they have early success with weight reduction of about 10–15 pounds and their energy levels and motivation are high, I begin to add mild exercise to their plan. This is usually a mild walking program. As the weight continues to decrease, I increase the time or speed of walking and as weight dramatically drops and energy levels begin to rise in a major way, I increase the overall exercise program and intensity of the activity. When the patient reaches their goal weight, they are now performing moderate or high intensity daily exercise and have incorporated both reduced calorie eating and higher calorie burning into their life.

Walking has been shown to be the activity of choice by the great majority of people who have lost over 30 pounds of weight and have kept it off for over a year. Walking is something that can be done almost anytime and anywhere. We can do it at home, in the neighborhood, at work, school, and the mall. We can do it with our pet or alone on a treadmill. You can combine other activities with your walking. I prefer to walk daily on my treadmill and watch my tablet in front of me to learn about new medical information, business information, or just fun reading. I can even watch the evening news while walking on my treadmill. With the power of electronic devices and the internet we can listen to our favorite music or podcasts about topics of interest while we walk. Many people tell me they don't walk because it's boring. With an iphone, ipod, or any portable device you can listen, learn, or party while you walk. With online educational programs and downloads, you could enhance your education on any topic and possibly work toward a degree while walking. I call these twofers. I get two important things done for the time it takes to do one. Two for One or twofers.

There are many other exercise programs that can lead to a leaner and fitter body and energetic lifestyle. Many of my clients love Zumba, Hot Yoga, dancing, spinning, swimming, or a variety of active sports they love to participate in. The point is to get off the chair or couch and build your activity level up to one hour every day. For those who think that an hour of physical activity a day is too much, remember it's only $1/24^{th}$ of your day. In comparison, the average person watches between 3 and 5 hours of TV daily. Taking care of your body is surely worth one hour each day. If nothing else, stick a treadmill or stationary bicycle in front of the TV. The tendency to regain weight if you are engaged in an hour of activity a day is markedly reduced. With the advent of motion monitors such as the FitBit and dozens of other similar devices, it's easy to see just how much activity you are performing each day. These devices talk to your computer or smart phone and can log your recorded daily activity alongside your daily calorie count. This type of monitoring gives you a real time log of your daily achievement both during your weight loss phase and in your weight maintenance phase. I use a simple inexpensive FitBit and link it to my cellphone which has the MyFitnessPal app on it. I track my daily calories and food intake on the MyFitnessPal app and my FitBit app sends my activity log automatically to the other app. At the end of the day, I know exactly where I stand with regard to my healthier lifestyle. By knowing and tracking this information, it's easier to set goals and make adjustments to our lifestyle.

As a physician, I recognize that not everybody can perform the typical exercises. Our weight, health conditions, diseases, and disorders play a large role in our ability to exercise. I have patients who are unable to walk for various reasons. I prescribe other types of physical activity for them. In extreme cases, the only exercise a patient can achieve is light chair exercises, but these are helpful in contributing to overall improvement in fitness, weight, and health. I'm asked many times which exercises are best for weight loss and weight loss maintenance. The answer is all exercise. They are usually asking whether aerobic exercise or resistance training is best. Both are important. I recommend daily moderate aerobic activity such as brisk walking, swimming, cycling, or something that gets the heart rate up and sustains a higher heart rate for at least 20–30 minutes. I recommend resistance training as part of the exercise regimen at least 3 days a week. I'm not talking about power lifting unless you're interested in body building as you move toward your lean healthy weight. Light weight repetitious lifting utilizing both upper and lower body muscle groups and core body muscles is a great benefit to toning, thinning, defining, and increasing the body's metabolism. Something as simple as resistance band training is a great benefit for muscle mass improvement without bulking up. These bands can be used at home and are great for travelers. They can easily fit into a suitcase or travel bag. Most hotels have a small exercise room with a treadmill, bicycle, elliptical machine, and a weight lifting machine or small free weights. We really have no excuse not to get 30–60 minutes of physical activity daily above and beyond our normal daily routine. My coaches have studied physical exercise and health and are great at recommending and monitoring a client's exercise program. Having someone to be accountable to is of great benefit when it comes to exercise. Call a friend or co-worker to take walks with. Knowing that someone else is going to join us is a great motivator for showing up even when we would rather not. Take the hint from the Nike Corporation . . . "Just Do It"!

THE MENTAL PLAN

Dr. Sklare, a renowned psychologist who has assisted my weight loss clinic in providing cognitive therapy to my patients says . . . "You can't change your weight until you change your mind". This is very true. There are a multitude of mental blocks that get in the way of our losing weight. How we perceive the process of losing weight, how we see food in our lives and the meaning we give it, how other emotional issues relate to our eating patterns, and even our personality type play a significant role in our resistance to losing weight. Weight loss deals with reducing food, increasing activity, learning to control our thoughts and our minds, and treating the disease process when necessary. People go on diets, lose some weight and then rapidly regain the weight. This cycle goes on over and over and even has a name for it . . . Yo-Yo Dieting. Up and down goes the weight and then we blame the diet because it failed, only to attempt the next latest diet fad or craze once again. Without focusing on the "Why" of our eating behavior, it will be impossible to keep the weight off. This mental component is as significant as the genetic and biochemical component I spoke of earlier. Without understanding how our brain and mind work when it comes to eating and overeating, we are destined to stay fat. A solid cognitive/behavior psychological program is needed in the weight loss process.

I know that when I say that a comprehensive treatment plan is needed, everyone thinks, "I don't have time or money to go to a psychologist or psychiatrist every week to change my thinking. The good news is that you don't have to. The program that we use in our clinic is called the InnerDiet by Dr. Sklare. This program will inform you with the psychological reasons you may overeat and provide a specific program designed for each person to guide them through the changes in thinking necessary to beat the obesity problem. The overeating screening survey gives each person a clear picture of why they eat too much. The self-guided, self-administered tutorial program covers the six major psychological reasons why people overeat and struggle to lose weight even while on a proper eating and exercise program. These reasons are Commitment, Discomfort, Inner Control, Perfectionism, Secondary Gain, and Stress Eating. Ninety-five percent of patients who take the initial profile questionnaire score high in one of the main areas. Eighty percent score high in at least two of the areas, and 60% score high in three of the areas. This data certainly suggests that our emotions are another major player in why we find it difficult to lose weight and keep it off. The program creates a strong awareness of our underlying psychological eating behaviors and provides a workbook to assist each person in retraining their mind to better deal with the issues. When combining a psychological treatment to our medical treatment and diet and exercise protocols, we have seen a tremendous increase in both short and long term success of our patients in losing the weight and maintaining a leaner body. Obesity and weight problems are complex and a comprehensive approach is required to get a person to their optimal weight and then assisting them in keeping it off indefinitely.

Every day in my practice, I talk with patients who struggle with stress eating, the discomfort of dieting, the ability to control their thoughts, and staying committed to eating a lower calorie, healthier meal plan. They want so badly to improve their looks, their health, and their lives. Getting someone to understand and believe that they can actually make it to their goal weight and stay there is the most difficult thing that I do every day. Combining cognitive and behavioral changes with the rest of the program can make the difference between losing a few pounds and losing all of the excess pounds. Being mentally in control and mindfully stronger is a powerful tool in the battle against weight gain and obesity. Let go of your mental blocks and accept the full treatment of overweight and obesity and you will make rapid and lasting strides toward living lean for the rest of your life.

THE MEDICAL PLAN

Our bodies are all different. Some people remain thin their entire lives no matter how and what they eat. Others gain and hold weight easily and rapidly. Still others bounce up and down in weight going on and off of dietary plans every few months. As previously discussed, we now know that our genetic tendencies play a big role in how we respond to our environment. The type of foods we prefer, and the signals that tell us we are hungry or that we're full are programmed into our chromosomes. The resultant chemistry of our body then works to determine our metabolic rate, our stomach to brain signaling mechanisms, our sense of satiety, and which foods seem to satisfy us most. There are a wide variety of medical conditions that promote weight gain and excess calorie consumption. These conditions fall into several categories that I define as:

1. Carbohydrate Sensitivity

2. Metabolic Syndrome

3. Hormonal Imbalance

4. Food Hypersensitivities

5. Medications

6. Sleep Disorders

7. Emotional Eating

There is treatment for each of these medical issues. Being able to control, stop, or manage these conditions is critical to achieving lasting weight loss. I have hundreds of patients who have had a medical disorder from one of these categories. Once the condition has been diagnosed and treated, they begin to lose weight when they were unable to lose more than a couple of pounds in their entire adult lives. It has been tremendously rewarding to work with patients who have tried every diet, supplement, and gimmick to try to lose weight and when properly diagnosed and treated the weight begins to drop off. A recent patient of mine with carbohydrate sensitivity was treated with medication, diet, and supplements to reduce her sensitivity and she has lost over 60 pounds. She is now full of energy and sees life from an entirely different perspective. The most weight she had lost on any previous diet was about 12 pounds, which rapidly came back. This was not magic and she still had to be very diligent with the treatment plan, but the results were self-motivating and self-sustaining. She now has a plan to work and live fully as a thin woman for the remainder of her new healthier life.

CARBOHYDRATE SENSITIVITY

This condition doesn't have a diagnosis code and won't be found in the medical literature, but I feel that it is a major cause of weight gain today. Highly processed and sugar rich foods in our American diet have overstimulated the eating centers and associated biochemistry in our brains and driven us to eat carbohydrates (sugar-based foods) at a greater frequency and higher volume than past generations have. Calorie dense carbohydrate foods mixed with high calorie fat is like a pleasure drug to the brain. The worst foods for this are the fried carbohydrates such as French Fries and chip snacks. Fried pastries such as donuts work the same way to create high levels of cravings for more of the same food. Recent data shows that these foods stimulate receptors in the brain in much the same way that other addictive substance do. Nicotine, narcotics, alcohol, and amphetamines also stimulate similar receptors in the brain and create a feeling of pleasure. As more of the addictive substance is taken into the body, the craving and desire for more intensifies and drives us to ingest additional substances. This desire for increased carbohydrates is a soft addiction. Ask any person with this disorder if they can eat a single chocolate chip cookie. The answer is usually, "I don't stop until the package is gone". Carbohydrate sensitivity can be discovered through listening to the eating history of a patient along with diagnostic testing which can show elevated triglycerides, increased fasting insulin levels, and sometimes slightly high blood glucose and hemoglobin A1c levels.

These patients do not have the official diagnosis of diabetes. However, without treatment this condition can lead to the future onset of diabetes. I begin treatment of this condition with a low carbohydrate diet consisting of a total daily carbohydrate intake of less than 100 grams. I like to increase protein intake to around 100 grams and keep their fat intake around 20–25 percent of total calories a day made up of healthier fats. This comes to about 1200 calories daily. The diet requires eating every 2.5 to 3 hours starting within one hour of awakening. I recommend specific portion controlled meal replacements of between 100 and 160 calories each to be eaten between any prescribed meals. Eating at these intervals keeps the body from sensing hunger and avoids the feeling of deprivation. I prescribe metformin 500mg twice daily to be taken with the small breakfast meal and the evening meal. This medication increases the body's sensitivity to its own insulin. In cases where marked overeating sessions is a problem, I will also use an appetite suppressant such as Diethylpropion or Phentermine to reduce overall appetite. Once control of appetite is accomplished through the diet, a greater amount of fat is being burned through lipolysis and the production of ketones for fuel, the appetite suppressants can be used to a much lesser extent. For the first time in a long time, these patients start to see real weight loss in a consistent manner. Once the weight loss has continued and about 10 pounds have been lost, I institute a mild daily exercise plan. The goal is to slowly increase the time and intensity of the exercise so that as the weight goes down the activity level goes up. I advise my patients that adding in any sweets, snacks, or carbohydrates not on the plan will reverse the preferential fat burning and that it will take about 3 days for the body to convert back to using fat as its primary fuel source. During this program designed to break the carbohydrate sensitivity, I stay in close contact with the patients through monthly visits, phone, email, or texts to answer questions and promote accountability. This treatment protocol works extremely well and with added psychological counseling, the patient will learn how to prevent the weight from returning when they complete the weight loss phase of the program.

Once at their goal weight and if insulin levels and glucose levels are in normal ranges, I will stop the medications. The appetite suppressants can be used on an intermittent basis for certain days when eating temptation occurs such as birthdays, holidays, and other special events. If the patients find themselves eating an increased amount of carbohydrates and gaining pounds in the future, they are instructed to contact me immediately. This is an emergency and if control is not regained quickly, they will go on to re-gain all of the weight lost and reverse the metabolic stability back to its detrimental status. The most important thing that I can impress upon my patient is that this is a life-long disorder, but that it can be well controlled with this therapy. In the maintenance phase, we are able to re-introduce foods back into the diet including certain carbohydrates, but in smaller quantities and with less frequent consumption.

Reversing carbohydrate sensitivity and being able to dramatically reduce fat and weight from the body, adds years to a person's life, and more importantly adds much more life to the additional years. This process of carbohydrate reduction can also reverse or delay the onset of diabetes for years to come. This is not easy, but every successful patient will tell me that the benefits received from the program far exceed any downside from the changes they've made. I have yet to find anyone who could not stay with the program, if they honestly were willing to do the work. There is no magic in this, but the implementation of sound treatment protocols and ongoing follow-up is necessary. I also have coaches in my practice that stay in touch with the patients throughout the program and beyond. Learning to reduce their total glycemic load and eat healthier low glycemic index foods will allow them to stay at their desired weight. These carbohydrate sensitive individuals are learning to retrain their body and mind to control their weight and health indefinitely. They will be able to live lean and long with an exciting, energetic life.

Glycemic Index is a numeric index that ranks carbohydrates based on how fast they are converted to glucose (sugar) within the body

Glycemic Load is a number that allows practical application of Glycemic Index to our diet. It is the Glycemic Index of a food times the net carbohydrates in a serving of food. It measures both quality and quantity of carbohydrate ingestion

METABOLIC SYNDROME

Metabolic Syndrome is a group of conditions that occur together in the body. They include high blood pressure, increased blood sugar levels, excess body fat (especially around the waist), and abnormal cholesterol and lipid levels. A major problem with this syndrome is that it leads to a very high risk of heart attack and stroke along with a strong risk for diabetes. These multiple conditions tend to come together in a genetic package. The conditions are associated with obesity and they each tend to negatively drive the other disorders. The weight gain increases blood pressure and lipid problems. These, in turn, provide biochemical changes that make diabetes more likely. A cycle of weight gain and progression of the conditions continues and the abdomen or belly becomes larger and larger. This abnormal accumulation of fat tissue takes on a life of its own producing inflammatory substances and hormones that perpetuate the problem.

Most physicians will treat the disorder by prescribing medication for each and every condition that comes with the disorder. Patients with metabolic disorder will take between 3 and 10 medications to control the blood pressure, cholesterols, blood sugars, and other disorders arising from the syndrome. The true treatment for this disorder is substantial weight loss and an increase in physical activity. Unfortunately, when people get to the point where they are dramatically overweight and they have difficulty moving around, it seems impossible for them to reverse the cycle and get back to a state of reasonably good health. It is possible to reverse the syndrome, but it requires aggressive intervention. Going on a short term diet will not fix the problem. A thorough review of the person's current eating, sleep and work habits as well as lifestyle will assist in designing a program that can help control and reverse the Metabolic Syndrome. As with carbohydrate sensitivity, these patients develop high insulin levels and cravings for sweets and unhealthy foods. They routinely overeat since the mechanisms that control hunger are altered by the excess fat tissue and its resultant release of toxic and detrimental substances into the bloodstream.

In order to reverse the syndrome, a dramatic change in the diet is required. For these patients, the goal is to reduce fat tissue in the body which in turn will reduce inflammatory processes and allow the normal functions of the body to return. My goal is to be able to reduce the amount of medications that the patient takes and to get them leaner so that they can begin an active exercise plan. Almost all of these people will tell me that they feel their appetite is out of control and that they are not satisfied with even a large meal.

I place these patients on a simple but rigid eating plan which eliminates shopping for food, preparing food, and cooking food. They have choices in their food selections, but they are all chosen from a predetermined list of portion controlled meal replacements. During this first month they will eat seven times a day or about every 2 to 2 and ½ hours while awake. Each snack meal, as I call them, will consist of about 15 grams of protein and about 8–12 grams of carbohydrate and 1–3 grams of fat. These very good tasting snack meals will provide about 900 calories a day. This is a mildly ketogenic diet and rapidly causes fat to be used as the prime fuel source for the body. The snack meals consist of shakes, bars, cookies, oatmeal, chips, and a wide variety of other mini-meals. These patients typically lose about 15 pounds of fat in the first month. Depending on the amount of weight to be lost, this will range between 10 and 20 pounds. This rapid and consistent fat reduction is very motivating and can begin to change the blood pressure, blood sugar, and insulin levels in dramatically positive ways. It is not unusual to have to lower medications for blood pressure and blood sugars in just the first month. At the beginning of the second month, the patient can continue with the seven snack meals alone or move to a program with 5 snack meals and one lean and green real food meal daily. Weight loss continues and at this point the addition of mild to moderate physical activity is a must.

My coaches assist with this education. I also have patients track their activity with a FitBit or pedometer. Daily self-monitoring is necessary to be able to keep a proper focus on the task. I have the patient keep track of both food intake and physical activity. I also have them work through a cognitive/behavior change program that will give them insight into their current eating issues and help them to change their thinking about food, eating, and weight in general. By aggressively tackling the Metabolic Syndrome disorder, a person can actually reverse elevated blood pressure, diabetes, high lipids and cholesterol, and eliminate the large belly and pool of fat that is negatively contributing to and perpetuating this disorder. A lean look and a clean check-up from the doctor is a great reward for going through the treatment plan to solve the disorder of Metabolic Syndrome.

HORMONAL IMBALANCE

This is a series of disorders that can affect both men and women. However, women seem to be effected at a much higher rate. Having the proper amount of hormones is crucial to proper growth, having energy, and being able to stay active and keep weight at optimal levels. I see many teenage girls with weight issues, many of which are caused by hormone imbalances. The most common abnormal hormone issue in adolescent women that leads to obesity is called Polcystic Ovarian Syndrome or PCOS. These girls gain weight rapidly after reaching puberty and have no or very irregular periods along with abnormal hair growth on the face and body. The symptoms vary and some girls present with only mild symptoms and the major complaint being rapid and uncontrolled weight gain. They are typically told that they eat too much and are lazy. However, the problem is created by the hormone imbalance. In these girls, the ability to control weight is a major issue. The underlying cause of this syndrome is unknown, however there does seem to be a family link to the disorder implicating a genetic factor. The ovaries develop cysts and the production of female and male hormones is altered. There is a larger percentage of male hormone being produced in the young woman than should be. This leads to the irregularity of periods, abnormal hair growth, excess acne, and some scalp hair loss. Symptoms can be variable among women. One common trait is that insulin levels are typically quite high. This will lead to excess appetite and dramatic fat production in some patients. Current treatment involves lowering the body's resistance to insulin and achieving sustained weight loss. The insulin resistance is an underlying problem and makes these young women's bodies very resistant to losing weight. They are also carbohydrate sensitive, most likely because of the high insulin levels and resultant craving for sugar-based foods.

The treatment of this disorder is focused on reversing the insulin resistance. Therefore, I start these patients on Metformin and adjust the medication dose upward to its maximum safe level. I also use a restricted carbohydrate diet and increase protein intake. Mild exercise to begin with is necessary, but the main focus is on dietary changes and eating control. I do find that appetite suppression helps greatly and use the appetite suppressant medication in girls over 14 years of age. Close follow-up and evaluation is required since there are many psychological issues that develop in teenagers who are obese and "different" from their peers. Monitoring blood sugar levels, hormonal levels, and parameters like lipids and cholesterol are important for long term management. When weight is reduced and insulin levels drop, menstrual periods become more regular and many of the symptoms resolve. The disorder is not cured but rather placed in remission. Some of the my greatest rewards in medicine have come from helping these young ladies re-take control of their bodies and live a happier more normal and leaner life.

THYROID DISORDERS

Hormones produced by the thyroid gland influence nearly all of the metabolic processes in the body. Disorders of this small gland in the front of our neck can be associated with dramatic weight changes and body function abnormalities. The thyroid gland can have a disorder of excess hormone production as well as disorders of diminished thyroid hormone production. Low levels of thyroid hormone production lead to a slowing down of the body. Heart rate is lower as is body temperature and the ability to burn calories. Weight gain is common with low thyroid function. Common symptoms of low thyroid levels include menstrual irregularities, constipation, depression, dry skin and dry hair with hair loss, fatigue, cold temperature intolerance, unexplained weight gain or trouble losing weight, and a slow heart rate. This disorder is more common among women but is also seen in men. Without spending a great deal of time on the causes of these disorders, it is important for every person with excess fat tissue and weight loss difficulties to be adequately tested for thyroid disease. Controversy exists over the optimal treatment levels of low thyroid among different physician groups, but I treat patients for the elimination of symptoms and monitor their progress closely to be sure that the optimal levels of hormone for each patient is achieved. With this hormonal disorder, there is a wide range of symptoms and variability in the degree of thyroid dysfunction. I have patients with classic symptoms and signs of low thyroid yet have been told by other physicians that their blood test is normal and that they have no problem. In these cases which are considered sub-clinical hypothyroidism, I believe that we are missing mild or early low thyroid problems. More aggressive evaluation and monitoring is called for as a mild adjustment of the thyroid level will make a dramatic effect on the health and well-being of the patient.

It is important when treating hypothyroidism (low thyroid function) that the condition not be over-treated or treated without ongoing monitoring. Overly aggressive treatment of the low thyroid problem can lead to creation of an excess thyroid state which is also dangerous to the patient. Low thyroid can be treated quite simply with thyroid hormone supplementation. I prefer the natural thyroid preparations since they contain amounts of both the active thyroid hormones, T3 and T4. Most doctors use only T4 preparations since the body does convert the T4 into T3. There are some vitamin and mineral deficiencies that can affect the conversion of T4 to T3. This must be checked in patients who are not responding properly to thyroid treatment. Once a person with low thyroid function is properly treated, previous resistance to weight loss can be rapidly eliminated. When I evaluate a patient for potential thyroid disease, I order labs that check TSH (thyroid stimulating hormone), T4 (thyroxine), T3 (triiodothyronine), thyroid antibodies, and in some cases Reverse T3 which is an ineffective form of T3.

Mainstream medical recommendations are to screen for thyroid disorders with a single TSH test and to repeat if abnormal to verify that it has not been affected by another recent illness. The TSH level itself can be altered by obesity and this must be taken into consideration when deciding when and how to treat thyroid disease. Though testing of TSH levels may certainly pick up the majority of patients with thyroid function problems, I and other physicians believe that many patients are being left untreated for a condition that is negatively affecting their life. Evaluation of thyroid lab tests and treatments are currently being undertaken to see if changes in current medical practice are needed to better diagnose and treat thyroid disorders. The major point of this discussion is to make patients aware that thyroid dysfunction can be a major obstacle to reversing obesity, improving energy, and living a thinner more vibrant life. It's worth getting a thorough thyroid test as part of an obesity, weight gain evaluation.

LOW TESTOSTERONE

Testosterone is the predominant sex hormone in men, but is also produced and is important in women. In looking at testosterone function in men it is important to understand that this hormone plays a larger role than just sexual desire and function. Testosterone is important for the development of all male sexual characteristics such as muscle size, voice deepening, penile and testicular size, hair patterns and sex drive. It is also important in bone strength, weight maintenance, depression, glucose metabolism, blood pressure, and heart disease. There are ongoing studies regarding testosterone and these disorders. Many feel that a decline in testosterone levels after age 30 is normal and should not be seen as a medical condition. Lately, the treatment of men with a variety of degenerative symptoms such as fatigue, decreased sexual desire and function, weight gain, depression, bone loss, and irritability has become more standard by utilizing testosterone supplementation.

There is considerable controversy in this arena. However, I believe that if hormone levels are low and symptoms are present, it is imperative to utilize appropriate treatment to enhance the life of my patient. With any treatment, proper diagnosis and long term follow up evaluation of the treatment is required and treating to appropriate response is advised. Good medical care never over-treats this disorder, but optimizes the hormone level for each individual. Standard total testosterone levels for men drop from age 30 to 100 in a very steady progressive pattern. Does this mean it is normal? Dropping testosterone levels is a typical pattern of aging men, but if symptoms with these lowering levels occur, which usually happens, then appropriate supplementation should be implemented. Symptoms of low testosterone include decreased muscle mass, increased body fat, fatigue, lack of sexual desire, irritability (grumpy old man syndrome), and increased risk for cardiovascular disease, diabetes, and other metabolic problems.

Testosterone supplementation can be given through the topical administration of a gel, cream or patch. It can also be given by an injection of long acting testosterone, and by pellet insertion with slow dissolving pellets placed under the skin. Close attention to the prostate gland and Prostate Specific Antigen levels (PSA), along with blood counts are important. Testosterone can increase the production of red blood cells which if high enough can cause problems. Testosterone supplementation has gotten a bad name due to the overuse by professional athletes and body builders in their attempt to make the body do things it's not normally made to do. If you are low in testosterone, then supplementing with this hormone to a normal and more optimal level can make a tremendous difference in your overall well-being and health. Proper treatment allows energy levels to rise, fat to be more easily reduced, sexual drive and function to be enhanced and the lack of motivation and loss of drive to be resolved.

TESTOSTERONE THERAPY IN WOMEN

Women also make testosterone, though in much smaller quantities than men. The primary sex hormones of females are estrogens and progesterone. The ovaries and adrenal glands make testosterone in women and after age 20 the levels begin to drop. Controversy exists as to whether women should receive supplementation with testosterone. Some data suggests that in women with premature menopause due to surgical removal of the ovaries, replacement of sex hormones, estrogen and progesterone and possibly small amounts of testosterone will maintain sexual desire and function. Current areas of women's health where testosterone therapy is being considered is in keeping bones strong and healthy after menopause, managing pain levels, and preserving cognitive health. The final answers on these benefits are not available at this time. My recommendation is that if you are postmenopausal with symptoms relating to hormone insufficiency, then evaluation and possible treatment with appropriate hormone supplementation including small amounts of testosterone may be significantly beneficial to alleviate the symptoms. The FDA has not approved testosterone therapy in women, although this does not restrict physicians from using it in this manner if the benefits outweigh the risks of treatment and the rationale for using it is well documented.

ADRENAL GLAND DYSFUNCTION

Our adrenal glands produce several hormones that effect our metabolism and how our body responds to stress. The adrenal gland produces cortisol which helps regulate metabolism and our stress response. It also produces aldosterone which regulates our fluid balance and helps control blood pressure. Other hormones are produced in this gland including adrenalin which is a fast acting hormone that allows our body to quickly respond to stress and danger. The cortisone type hormones from the adrenal gland regulate how our body converts fat, protein, and carbohydrates into energy. Excess cortisol can contribute to excess fat deposition in the body. The extreme of the excess cortisol is called Cushing's Syndrome. When cortisol and aldosterone are extremely low, this disorder is known as Addison's Disease. These two disorders are at the polar extremes of adrenal gland function. It is now thought that a wide variety of adrenal gland dysfunctions may occur leading to a multitude of negative symptoms such as fatigue, weight gain, irritability, and fluid retention disorders.

Adrenal fatigue is a new term that describes decreased function of the gland. It is felt that due to our high stress lives, poor sleep patterns, and poor diets, the adrenal gland can burn out over time. In its effort to combat day in and day out stress, the gland overproduces cortisol which leads to increased appetite and fat production. When the gland becomes "worn out", then generalized fatigue, irritability, forgetfulness, and symptoms that slow down the body and mind occur. Treatment is designed to restore normal adrenal gland function. It includes eliminating as much daily stress as possible, eating a very healthy diet of lower fat, lower carbohydrate foods and taking some support supplements that enhance the body and adrenal gland function. When the adrenals are functioning optimally, the body responds to our attempt at fat reduction in a much improved way. Reducing stress and getting adequate sleep is a key to improving the function of our adrenal glands. Sleep is important for our metabolic functions to perform at peak levels. I've had many patients with obstructive sleep apnea lose weight when the apneic episodes are improved or resolved. I believe that one of the reasons is that the enhanced oxygenation and resultant sleep supports our organs like the adrenal gland and also assist our mind in managing stress throughout the daytime. The important consideration is to be mindful of the negative effects of stress on the hormonal systems and that this will lead to marked increase in signaling for the production of fat. One of the components of our program involves dealing with the mind and working to reduce the stress that leads to overeating in up to 85% of obese people. If you're struggling with weight loss, get evaluated for adrenal dysfunction as well as seek assistance to better handle or eliminate stress in your daily life. This alone may be an answer to getting lean and staying lean for the rest of your life.

FOOD HYPERSENSITIVITY

We have known for decades about acute food allergies. These are the dangerous allergies that everyone knows about such as peanut allergies, strawberry allergies, and similar rapid detrimental responses to certain foods that some people develop. These allergies are caused by antibodies in our blood that violently respond to the offending food in the allergic person. These antibodies are known as IgE antibodies. They cause hives, itching, tissue swelling and can even block our airways due to the swelling in severe cases. They require aggressive and quick treatment. There is another type of food allergy that involves a much slower and less acute process. It is regulated by the response of a different antibody known as IgG. This antibody deals with chronic sensitivity to a substance entering our body, in this case a food. Over time, the slow reaction to certain foods will cause a low grade inflammation in our intestinal lining and this inflammation can cause microscopic leaks that allow toxins from our intestines back into our blood stream. This disorder is currently called "Leaky Gut Syndrome". This disorder will cause a multitude of digestive symptoms, but will also cause general symptoms in the body such as fatigue, irritability, chronic pain, weight gain, unusual dietary preferences, and sleep problems. This low grade toxic process alters our body's metabolism and its ability to properly function with regard to many signaling mechanisms including hunger and satiety.

Patients with these food sensitivities will present with a list of symptoms that have been previously diagnosed as depression, fibromyalgia, irritable bowel syndrome, chronic fatigue, and a host of other chronic conditions. While these other disorders exist and may even co-exist with leaky gut syndrome, uncovering this disorder can allow for enhanced digestion, elimination of fatigue and the ability to exercise and eat a proper diet that will not irritate the intestinal tract and the rest of our sensitive systems. I have many patients that have told me after treating these food sensitivities that they have not felt so good nor have they been able to function so well in many years. These food sensitivities can come from any food source and the more these foods are ingested, the greater the allergic response becomes.

Once the specific foods that cause the inflammation are known, elimination of the most severe offending foods and rotation in smaller quantities and eating frequencies of the less irritating foods will allow the leaks in the gut to heal and eliminate the toxicity to the body. After time, some of the foods that produce mild to moderate sensitivity can be re-introduced in the diet in limited quantities without causing any problems. The testing for these food sensitivities is not common among current practicing physicians, but this information is being disseminated to doctors at medical meetings and in the scientific literature. I also have noticed dramatic weight loss in patients once the foods they are sensitive to have been eliminated from the diet or diminished significantly. Improvement in digestion and the body's ability to process foods is markedly enhanced and the symptoms of constipation, diarrhea, and abdominal pain become a thing of the past. If you continually struggle with abdominal and digestive symptoms, have persistent fatigue, and just can't seem to lose any weight with dieting, I urge you to get to a physician who will evaluate you for IgG food sensitivities and Leaky Gut Syndrome. Your health depends on it and your ability to function at a higher level requires a proper diet that avoids these detrimental foods. You can lose the weight, get the nutrients you require, eliminate chronic debilitating medical issues with a change in diet to foods that your body doesn't fight.

WEIGHT GAIN FROM MEDICATIONS

I encounter patients every day that have struggled with weight gain and have never found a reason why. When they are questioned, I often find that the weight gain began in association with some other disorder. When the other disorder was diagnosed, they were placed on medication to control the condition. Little did these patients know that the very medication that was helping with the other disease was causing weight gain, obesity, and in some cases diabetes. There are many medications that have weight gain as a common side effect or adverse reaction. Physicians tend to downplay this since they are primarily interested in treating a disease state and do not consider the weight gain a disease state in itself. In rare cases of certain severe disorders, weight gain may be a reasonable acceptable side effect if the patient has no other alternatives for treatment. In most cases, however, alternative therapies that lead to less or no weight gain do exist.

Certain high blood pressure treatments will cause weight gain by slowing the body down. Beta Blockers are notorious for this. In the treatment of migraine headaches, seizure disorders, chronic nerve pain, and spinal disorders, many medications cause significant weight gain. In the area of depression therapy, a large number of medications cause increase in appetite and resultant weight gain. Even nerve pills and narcotic pain pills reduce our energy output and cause excess fat accumulation. A list of medications that cause weight gain and are routinely used for typical medical conditions is provided below. If you are taking any of these medications and have experienced the common weight gain phenomenon with them, ask your physician or health care provider to look for an alternative therapy without this complication. It may take some searching and trials of different medications, but in the long run you should be able to treat one disease without causing a second one, in this case obesity.

We get a history of current medications that our patients take who enter our weight management clinic. It is quite typical to find that these struggling weight losers are taking medications that make it difficult for their body to function in a way that will allow for the excess fat to be burned off. It is truly amazing when an adjustment in a medication allows for both the treatment of the primary disease such as high blood pressure and the ability to lose weight. Often, significant weight loss leads to lowering of the blood pressure and even the ability to go off some or all of their blood pressure medications. We have entered a time in the practice of medicine where it is common for doctors to treat one condition with a medication and when the side effects of that particular medication occur a second medication is given to treat the side effects. Over time, patients with several medical conditions can end up on 10 to 15 different prescription medications used to treat the disorders and the negative effects of the treatment of the disorder. The problem with taking medications that cause weight gain or the resistance to weight loss is a simple problem to correct. It is rare that a substitute therapy cannot be found.

Ask your physician or primary provider to review your medications to see if a change or adjustment can be made to assist with your treatment of the disease of obesity. If you don't get a satisfactory response from your doctor, it's time to get a second opinion. My belief is that the two most prevalent and significant problems that patients can have are smoking and obesity. If a physician won't give attention to assisting a patient with elimination of these two medical hazards, then you need a new physician who is interested in preventing disease primarily and managing disease secondarily. The current healthcare system is focused on treating disease. Our goal should be preventing disease. Unfortunately, both insurance companies and patients are not very interested at this time in prevention, requiring out of pocket payment for high quality preventive care. Everyone gives lip service to prevention, but very few are actually digging deep into preventing disease with each and every patient visit. Treating obesity cannot be handled like treating a sore throat or flu syndrome. However, most patients and doctors see it this way. Commercial diet programs also treat obesity in a limited way. They treat the problem until some weight is lost and if it returns, then treat it again. This is not for you. You want to put obesity into remission and live a life of controlled weight with a low-fat body. Find a healthcare provider who will work as a partner with you in the long term treatment of excess fat accumulation and assist you in preventing the need for multiple medications, some of which will confound the ability to lose weight. Set a plan today to have medications reviewed and help you doctor help you to drop the unwanted pounds.

SLEEP APNEA

This disorder is very prevalent in our society. It is made worse by the epidemic of obesity and is also a factor that can cause weight gain to be easier and more extreme. Our body and brain require adequate sleep for it to function properly. Sleep apnea prevents complete and restful sleep and dramatically reduces the restorative power of sleep. There are people that have obstructive sleep apnea and are thin. However, there is a direct correlation between increased body size and the development and severity of obstructive sleep apnea. When screening for sleep apnea, I consider body size, neck size, throat opening size, severity of snoring, daytime sleepiness symptoms, and sleep habits and patterns. If these signs point to the possibility of sleep apnea, then a sleep study is warranted. Many people with sleep apnea, who sleep with a partner, have been told by that partner that they stop breathing at times when they are asleep. This partner may have also noticed gasping for breath and a general pattern of poor sleep with the affected individual. Obstructive sleep apnea patients are not getting enough rest, and are not getting enough oxygen throughout the night. This negatively effects daytime energy levels, cognitive processes, and even our body's metabolic rate. I have many patients who have been diagnosed with obstructive sleep apnea. With proper treatment, they have felt much better during the daytime and have found that they have extra energy in their life to accomplish more at work and to even become more involved with exercise and hobbies.

It's also true that the reduction of body fat and weight can have a dramatic effect on the improvement and possible elimination of obstructive sleep apnea in patients. One of my patients comes to mind immediately. She lost over 100 pounds and was able to stop her nighttime CPAP machine (treatment for sleep apnea). She has not had to use the machine in the past several years after having attained and stayed near her goal weight. A repeat sleep study by her sleep specialist confirmed the resolution of the sleep apnea problem. I have many patients that have had these same results after weight loss. Treating obesity is the absolute best way to treat obstructive sleep apnea and treating obstructive sleep apnea is required to assist many patients to be able to lose weight effectively and consistently. If you are overweight by more than 30 pounds, snore, have daytime fatigue and sleepiness, and if anyone has ever noticed an unusual sleep pattern or breathing pattern during your sleep, be sure to schedule an appointment with you physician right away to discuss the possibility of obstructive sleep apnea. A simple questionnaire and check-up will confirm the possible existence of this severe medical disorder. You may learn that one of the major hurdles to your ability to get lean has been obstructive sleep apnea. Many other medical conditions can arise from this disorder such as hypertension, cardiovascular disease and lung disorders. Obstructive Sleep Apnea may also play a role in many other conditions. A new specialty of sleep medicine has developed over the past 15 years due to the severe nature of this disorder and the resultant complications in patients that have it.

EMOTIONAL EATING

Much of what I have talked about has been related to the physical and medical condition of obesity. Genetics, biochemistry, hormones, environment, sleep, medications, and addictive patterns all play strong roles in the obesity disorder. We can't change our genes but we can alter how our genes, body chemistry and hormones, and body signaling mechanisms work by altering our diet and physical activity. The science of epigenetics is the study of how our external environment effects the expression of our genes. What we eat, the toxins we encounter in our lives, and any other external factor that our body encounters can have an effect on the way our genes are turned on or turned off. Our ability to control what, when and why we eat, will help to reprogram our body's chemistry and may be able to adjust how our genes actually work in making us who we are.

This knowledge places a strong emphasis on the importance of our ability to take control of our eating. Being able to control our eating is the mental aspect of the disease of obesity. Our mind is extremely powerful and most of us don't give a second thought to how our mind works. We operate on patterns of behavior that we have established over many years. We behave in a way that has become comfortable for us. *Resistance* to our habits is not easy. Remember the discussion on *Resistance* and how it has a life of its own within our mind. We can overcome the evils of *Resistance* and we can change our habits. One of the most important things you can remember is that we as humans have been given the gift of choice and free will. We have minds that can be used to think. We generate a thought, which leads to an action, which over time becomes a habit, which develops into a behavior and then leads to a lifestyle that ultimately decides the trajectory of our entire life. Will we control the body we have or will it control us? Will we blame obesity on our genes and our "big bones", or will we take charge and create the body we want? All of the chapters to this point have explained the "how" to take charge and which appropriate actions are needed to lose weight. Unless we get our mind on board with our journey to thin and stay focused on the "why" underlying our desire to lose weight, our efforts will fail.

We all know that inside our head sits our brain, but it is our brain that creates our mind. I see the brain and mind as two separate and distinct entities in our body. The brain is the organ that is made up of billions of cells and trillions of connections with thousands of chemicals, transmitters, on-off switches, and electrical impulses. From all of that comes our ability to think and process the world around us. This processing capacity and function is our mind. The amazing thing is that our mind can actually alter and change the composition and even the structure of our brain. Studies have shown that someone who has depression, which is a biochemical disorder of the brain will think in an abnormal way. If this abnormal thinking pattern lasts long enough, the structure and composition of the brain will actually be altered. This can result in a permanent change in the brain. Have you ever known someone who was depressed their entire life no matter what treatment they received? I have seen hundreds if not thousands of patients with depression who have failed on every medication and every attempt at psychological therapy. I suspect that these patients fall into this category of having a permanent and negative alteration of the brain that has led to this long term condition. It is critical to be able to change how we think about weight, obesity, and its treatment. It is imperative to change our thought patterns about eating. When we have treated the mind for the obesity problem, then the other factors that affect our ability to control our weight can be managed much more easily.

Eighty-five percent of obese patients have some form of emotional eating behavior. This can occur with both positive and negative emotions. Food has become associated with emotional feelings. When these emotional feelings occur, we go into non-normal eating patterns. Our ability to break these old eating behaviors and habits through changing our cognitive patterns will provide a major breakthrough in the quest for living a leaner and healthier life. The big question is "How do I change my thinking"? The number one thing that must happen is to become aware that the thinking problem of emotional eating exists in you. Once you become aware of the emotional eating pattern, you can uncover the process that occurs and then work to change the habit through changing your thoughts. I realize that this sounds a bit weird, but hang with me. I will go through a process that can work for you. You will be able to know when the emotional eating pattern is coming on you and you will develop tools to use to learn to control the eating response to emotional stress.

A key component of changing our thinking so that we can change our action comes from self-awareness. All of us that have the obesity disorder know what it is like to mindlessly eat. Many of my patients sit in front of a television with a bag of chips or cookies only to end the program with an empty bag and don't even remember what the food tasted like. Being aware of our appetite and our hunger and the desire to act on it is extremely important to stopping the thoughtless eating pattern. How do we become more aware of our own body and mind? It's not as hard as one might think. In order to eat any food, the thought of eating must first arise. This can happen because we are truly hungry or because of some internal or external false signal, that makes us want to eat. If the signal is from real hunger, then eat an appropriate meal to supply the proper nutrition. If, however, the signal is from something else such as tension or stress or boredom, then we must learn to question the signal.

To do this we must stop and ask ourselves a series of simple questions. The first question is whether you are actually hungry. Next, ask yourself what is causing the signal to eat. Examples could be nervousness, fear, excitement, boredom, location, or even the person that you are with. We get many signals to eat from our environment. A good friend that always wants to meet at a coffee shop for a snack may later on signal the urge to eat something with a phone call or text. These signals become deeply anchored into our subconscious mind. We must use our conscious mind to assess the signals and then act differently. Once we raise the awareness of why we eat something to a level of consciousness, then we can make a better decision not to eat. I used to get up during a TV commercial and open the pantry door. I felt like a robot and didn't even think about why I was doing this. Over time when I would get up, I would stop and ask myself several questions. 1. "Am I hungry?" 2. "What is causing me to get up to search for food?" 3. "What else might I do to satisfy this urge?" Over time, I was able to control the cravings since I realized that these were false signals of hunger. The eating pattern had resulted in years of not even questioning the urges. You can also learn to ask a few simple questions that will more appropriately direct your behavior. The ability to use our conscious mind to decide to act or not act on an urge is what makes us human. Remember that you are human and have these choices. You are not a robot or just an instinctual animal following triggers and prompts.

Another psychological issue that confronts us in our weight loss effort is how we feel about the dieting process. Most of my patients see going on a reduced calorie eating plan as a punitive thing. "I've lived life eating anything and everything that I've wanted and now it's time to pay the price". The problem with this is that it focuses on negativity and only on a short term process. It's kind of like going to prison for a few months to atone for something bad that you've done. Only when you can change your thinking to view healthy eating as something that you want to do and get to do in order to have unlimited energy, a fit and leaner body (translate "sexy body" for many), and a life that is not bound by disease, pain, and inability to get around, will you enjoy the journey to thin. Even once you arrive at thin, you will see eating as the process you enjoy to keep your body and mind, both fit and active. You will be rewarded every day by living life this way. The mental and physical discomfort that you associate with the weight loss process can be reconditioned and turned into excitement and acceleration of your motivation.

Being able to change how we think about a process and re-program our minds to turn the past act of short term dieting into the lifetime act of eating well will allow you to create the body and life that you've only dreamed about in the past. Get excited to work on your mind at the same time that you are working on your body. One of the greatest understandings that we can come to is that we have the ability to change our thinking and our actions at any time. We have the ability to make life as good (or as bad) as we want it to be. It takes much more that a pep talk; but, ongoing positive self-talk and awareness of how we feel and why we feel that way can lead to an extraordinary life. This works with weight loss and weight maintenance and in every other area of our lives such as our relationships, careers, finances, and spirituality. By learning how to better operate our brain and improve our thought/response mechanism, we will live life as a shining example to those around us and enjoy every moment of our ride through life.

Some people see the weight loss process as an impossible feat. They have tried every diet plan, diet supplement and fad and gimmick. After these attempts, they have kept the weight on or even gained more. They feel that they are a failure. Here is an extremely important fact you must know. Failure is not a person, it is an event. We are not failures at anything. We can have a failed effort or activity. The great thing about going through a failed attempt at something is that we learn what doesn't work and can make changes so that another attempt can be more successful. As Thomas Edison said about his difficulties inventing the light bulb, "I have not failed, I've just found 10,000 ways that it won't work". When we have a failed attempt at weight loss, it's very important to understand the lesson. The way I went about it didn't work so I need to alter what I do to lose weight. I ask patients about past attempts to lose weight to see what they have learned about the process and themselves. Unfortunately, in many cases, the lesson has not been learned. That lesson is that losing weight and keeping it off is not about a short term low calorie diet. It's about a lifestyle change and the thinking process that brings that improved lifestyle into fruition. When you are truly serious about dropping the extra fat pounds and are ready to live life lean, then focus on improving the way you <u>think</u> about eating, food, nutrition, dieting, and exercise. These new cognitive skills will lead to a new way of losing weight. Your thoughts will lead to a purpose, which will move you toward actions, which will form new habits, decide your character and create your destiny. Subtle changes in your thinking about the way you eat will alter how much you eat and what you eat. This can establish new healthier and lower calorie eating habits that will lead you to becoming the person with the character that would not overeat or overindulge, thus leading to a new life. It all begins with changing your thinking.

Another psychological issue that affects our ability to lose weight is perfectionism. Many of us must have things exactly right or we will not move forward. It is all or nothing with us. We start a dietary regimen and for the first week we are strict and conform to the program without any mistakes or alterations. Along comes a Saturday evening social event and you give into a sweet indulgence of a slice of cheese cake. At this point, you become upset with yourself and decide that the diet is over. If I can't be perfect at it then I will not continue. This perfectionistic behavior pattern can sabotage us in our quest for a leaner body. If we think about it, we see that we have thrown the baby out with the bathwater. OK, we ate an extra 350 calories of a high carb dessert. The world didn't end. We didn't suddenly gain a pound or two. We ate something not on the program. The best thing to do now is to accept it, (hopefully you enjoyed the great tasting cheese cake) adjust your plan, and move forward. This might entail a little longer walk tomorrow. It might just mean that the morning brings a new day and the dietary program continues. If we become too hard on ourselves when we make a digression, then we are doomed to not succeed at the plan. We must learn to think and be more flexible.

I'm not saying that if you want to lose weight that you can digress from the plan all day, every day. This is not a weight reduction plan at all. This is denial. It is important to realize that situations come up when we need to adjust our plan and then move back to the plan as soon as possible. When I visit my mother's house, I know that she is going to have some delicious treat waiting for me. I know that I will not be able to say no to her, so I plan in advance to have a small slice of the confection and enjoy it with her. I make sure I plan for the additional calories by increasing my activity or by adjusting a meal later in the day or the next day. By thinking in advance of certain situations, it is possible to control the amount of calories you take in and not hold yourself to a level of accountability that no one can live up to. You will likely never fully correct the perfectionistic behavior, but you can learn to become a bit more flexible and allow yourself to continue on the journey to thin, even if a moment of temptation occurs.

There is a small percentage of people who suffer from the inability to lose weight for a very serious psychological reason. These patients are obese and continue to stay obese for secondary gain. You like most will wonder why someone would get a benefit from staying overweight. These patients are typically more than 100 pounds over their ideal weight. The obesity is a protective mechanism. We typically see this in people that are subconsciously wanting to avoid relationships, especially close relationships. They feel that by being obese they will not attract the attention of other people and more importantly will be able to avoid any close or intimate relationship. These patients have varying histories but a common component is verbal, physical, or sexual abuse. In many cases, the abuse was perpetrated by someone very close to them. They are hiding inside their grossly overweight body. The fat is a protective suit of armor for them. If you or someone you know suffers from this disorder, intensive psychological therapy to overcome it is usually required. Many of these patients will go through bariatric surgery only to lose a limited amount of weight and then rapidly put it back on. I've seen amazing long term results in these patients when they are able to open up about the pain they have experienced in their lives and to come to terms with the fact that the person who abused them is to blame and not them. If they can begin to trust other people again, the weight loss that occurs is truly incredible. When I encounter a morbidly obese individual that just can't lose the weight, I consider the possibility that a deep seated psychological problem exists. In this case, curing the mind will cure the obesity.

Lack of commitment is a major reason that individuals struggle with weight loss. Everyone who is overweight wants to be thinner. It's just that getting there is hard work and hard work takes a high level of commitment and persistence. It would be wonderful if one single concentrated effort would resolve the weight problem and cure obesity for the remainder of our lives. That just won't happen. Many people think that they lack discipline and that's why they don't lose the weight. I'm here to tell you that discipline and willpower play a much smaller role in weight loss than people think. All of my weight loss patients demonstrate willpower and discipline in many areas of their lives. Any person that holds a job has discipline. Getting up every morning and being at work on time requires effort and repetition. Raising children or staying in a relationship takes commitment, discipline, and willpower. We all have these characteristics and demonstrate them in areas that matter to us. I know, you are saying that weight loss matters. I would argue that even though you want to lose the weight, you have been unwilling to commit in the same fashion you commit to your job, your kids, or your partner. When you make the decision that losing excess weight is as important as those other three things, your level of focus and intensity toward losing weight will dramatically improve. You will see the discipline and willpower that already exists inside of you come out with a vengeance.

We are not lacking in the skills and abilities to lose the weight. We are lacking in the understanding of what is causing the weight problem and the lifetime consistency needed to put obesity into remission. My purpose in writing this book is to give you a greater understanding of what has caused you to have weight issues and what must be done on a daily basis to lose the excess weight and to maintain a leaner body for the rest of your life. A total effort that involves proper diet, regular exercise, learning how your mind operates is required. You must also learn how to reprogram some disempowering thinking that will move you toward becoming a thinner and more vibrant person. Commitment is an all or nothing concept. We are either working in the direction of thin or we are not. I'm not talking about minor setbacks. It requires a day to day, week to week, month to month, and year to year ongoing effort to control your own health. Commitment begins with a single decision that you will absolutely refuse to live life in an overweight, unhealthy body. Decision means to "cut away from". You are cutting away from living life as a fat person. You are cutting away from overeating. You are cutting away from the diseases that come from years of obesity. It's time to make that decision. Treating obesity is not like treating a cold. A week of change will not cure the obesity disease. Acceptance of true lifestyle change along with proper long term treatment will transform your body and your life. As Dr. Sklare says "You can't change your weight until you change your mind". Make that decision and get started today.

CHAPTER 9
LIVING LEAN, LIVING LONG, AND LIVING LIFE

You can now stop blaming yourself for the extra pounds that you have accumulated over the years. There are enough negative and bad things happening in our world that the last thing we need is to be our own worst critic. Each of us is here for a reason. Our life's purpose could be to be a mom or dad. It could be to help others learn or how to become successful in life. It might be that you are here to be an example for someone else. The bottom line is that we are all unique and we all have talents and we all have faults. We all make both good decisions and bad decisions. Your job now is to focus on the good in your life, the good things you have to offer, and the good things that are ahead of you. Losing weight and, in particular, excess fat tissue will allow you to function at your best capacity in accomplishing the things that you want and need to accomplish. Living life with a lean body will provide you with the energy and the strength to accomplish more in a single day than you might have thought possible in a week. Resolving your weight issue and conquering this problem that rests heavy on your mind every day of your life will free you to become who you have always believed deep inside that you could be. Learning how to break through the *Resistance* of serious weight loss will lead to breaking through *Resistance* in any area of your life. Achieving successful weight loss will create an ongoing drive for achievement in other areas of your life such as relationships, career, finances, spiritual endeavors, and fitness.

Being able to understand our body and our mind in a way that moves us toward our goal weight will continue and let us reach even deeper into who we are and why we do the things we do, both good and bad. Knowing that you are not alone in your weight loss struggle; and, that even though there are causes of your obesity that are out of your control, there are techniques and strategies that will allow you to reach your optimal weight and maintain it for the rest of your life. Our genetics are set, although new research indicates that some of our genes may soon be able to be turned on or off. Our biochemistry may create certain drives within us, but by changing both our physical and mental habits, we can alter the biochemistry of our body and mind. Our environment cannot be controlled by us, but how we involve ourselves in the environment can be totally controlled by us. We can decide how to eat, move and think. We are not drones being controlled by companies, advertisers, and the government. We are able to think for ourselves, act for ourselves, and make informed choices in every area of our daily lives including our food consumption. To lose weight you must begin with the end in mind.

Once we know what our true healthy weight should be, then setting a goal along with a daily action plan will allow us to know if we are making proper progress in the right amount of time. Goals are very important. I have many weight loss patients tell me that the goals they set seem meaningless and they struggle to hit even the easiest of goals. The problem is not in the goals, it's in the commitment, motivation, reasons, and drive behind losing weight. I've already covered many of these factors in this book. I am a goal setter. My son, Dave is a goal setter. Not until his middle twenties, did he see value in setting goals and plans to achieve them. I invited Dave to attend a weekend Goal Setting workshop, called "Creating Your Destiny" where he learned the correct way to set goals and how to break them down into actionable items and tasks to perform. During that weekend he dug deep into what he really wanted out of every area of his life. He worked hard to come up with what really mattered to him. This was the first time that he had actually focused and put significant time and effort on directing his own life. Many people say they have goals, but the truth is that most people spend more time planning a vacation than they do planning their lives. Losing weight, getting healthy, and becoming fit are worthy goals for every human. Spending time learning how to decide "why" we want to lose weight and "what to do" to lose weight will take some serious thought and work to develop.

After spending those 2 ½ days discovering what he wanted his life to look like and how to get there, Dave set out on his journey. One of his major goals was to get lean and fit. As a person whose job keeps him at a desk and a computer, he had gained over 80 pounds since leaving high school. Once he understood why he wanted to lose weight and get healthy, and had written a specific action plan to achieve his goal, he was able to drop those 80 pounds in about 6 months. He learned things he had never learned before. He began exercising which was something that he never did or wanted to do in his youth. He studied how specific physical activities along with proper eating skills allowed his body to burn fat and build lean tissue. By accomplishing this, he was able to understand other things about his life. He started to work on goals in other areas of his life such as business and finances. He set career goals that seemed impossible to achieve. He set goals in developing better relationships with his friends and associates, which ultimately led to finding his life's partner. Dave doesn't always hit his goals and on occasion backslides with weight and fitness. He understands that the disease of obesity will always be there and that staying dedicated to his original life goals can and does bring him back to a healthy state. The most important thing that he has learned is that he is the one that is in control of his body and that the fat genes, fat inducing chemistry, and quick easy high calorie foods in our environment can be overcome and put in their place.

You have this same ability. I will teach you how to go through an abbreviated process of deciding what you want with your health and body and then help you to design a plan to get there. The body you want and the life you want to live are up to you. Yes, you may need assistance from a doctor, dietitian, coach or trainer. Yes, you may need someone to hold you accountable as you proceed and progress. Yes, you will have missteps and backslides. You will meet *Resistance* head on and learn to break through it and to ultimately overcome it. Your ability to achieve what you want will build confidence, and power. This power will come into every aspect of your life. Let's take a look at how to establish worthy and realistic goals.

GOAL SETTING

Goals can be very powerful. However, the right goals for the right reasons are of greater significance. The first thing that must be determined is what you really want. Many of my patients come to me and when we ask them what they want to accomplish, they say things like, "I need to lose a few pounds", or "I want to feel better", or "I want to look better". These wishes are good but they are not empowering goals. For a goal to be powerful, it must be very specific. A goal must also be time specific. If we don't have a deadline to achieve something, it is unlikely that we will ever achieve it. One thing that I always ask myself when setting a goal is "How much by when". How much weight must I lose and when must I lose it is what is needed for a proper goal to be set. Many will argue that setting a goal to lose weight is not appropriate since it just takes a change in lifestyle. It is correct that adjustments in lifestyle including mental, eating and physical changes are necessary, but unless you have a time constrained specific focus, the overwhelming majority of people will dabble at the weight loss effort. I find that losing a specific amount of fat in a specific amount of time creates excitement, motivation, self-discipline, and new habits that can be built upon for additional improvement in weight and health.

Have you ever attended a sporting event? Of course, we all have. Have you ever attended a sporting event that wasn't played over a specific allotted time? Even non-timed sports events have endings which are determined by matches, innings, laps, or another time limiting factor. Have you ever attended a sporting event where the score was not kept or there were no goals to shoot at or achieve? No one would ever attend them and the participants in the sporting event would lose interest and would only perform at a lackluster pace. If there were no end result and no potential for victory, it would be boring and have no purpose. A while back, there was a trend in youth sports to not keep score since it was felt that competition had a negative effect on self-esteem and the learning of the game. This idea fell flat since the kids had no interest in the game and they kept score in their heads anyway, knowing that not keeping score was nothing more than practice. You don't want to practice at losing weight, you want to win the event of losing weight. You want to become a champion at losing weight.

Determining a specific weight goal that is healthy for you can be uncovered with a discussion with your healthcare provider. There are many scales and charts that are used to determine healthy weights. A BMI between 18 and 24 is considered a healthy range. For women, a weight of 100 pounds at 5 feet tall is considered ideal and adding 5 pounds to each inch over 5 feet tall would estimate ideal weight. An adult woman of 5 feet 6 inches would have an ideal weight of 130 pounds. Healthy ranges are typically within 10 percent of this ideal weight. For men, start with a weight of 106 pounds at 5 feet tall and add 6pounds per inch. A man who is 5 feet 11 inches tall would have an ideal weight of 172 pounds. A 10 % variance from this weight would be in the healthy range. This 10% variation accounts for age, body build type, and genetic variations from person to person. Once you have established your ideal weight and healthy range, you can set a goal. For a person who needs to lose over 100 pounds, setting a goal for their ideal weight may seem a bit daunting. In this case, a starter goal of say 30 or 40 pounds would be great. Once that goal is achieved another can be set. Once you know your goal weight, you need to set a timeline. I like realistic goals that make us stretch our ability. Setting a goal to lose 10 pounds in a month is a great stretch goal. Setting a goal to lose 10 pounds in a year will be boring and likely cause a loss of interest. On the other hand, setting a goal to lose 30 pounds in a month is not a good goal. It is unrealistic for 99% of people working to get thinner. A good goal example would be: "I am 10 pounds lighter on January 31", providing your goal was started on January 1.

Goals must be written. Keeping them in your head is a recipe for a failed attempt at weight loss. We have so much going on in our minds that it is unlikely that this goal will remain a priority if it remains a thought. By writing the goal down with pen and paper, it is many times more likely to be achieved. There is power in establishing written goals. Many studies have proven this over the years. Only 3–5% of people have written goals and that is exactly the percentage of people who are high achievers in our society. This is a clue. Success in anything leaves clues. Before you proceed any further, establish your WRITTEN goals for your weight loss journey. Here are some bullet points that will make this process fun and easy.

- Your weight loss goal must be specific

- Your weight loss goal must have an end date assigned to it

- Your weight loss goal must be written down

- Your weight loss goal must be realistic but a stretch

- Your weight loss goal should be written in the present tense:

"It is January 31ˢᵗ and I weigh 175 pounds"(10 pounds down from the month before at 185 pounds)

- Your weight loss goal must be in front of you daily (Put the goal on a card and put it on your bathroom mirror, the fridge, in your car, etc.)

- Your weight loss goal must have an action plan:

  "I walk 10,000 steps daily and eat 1500 calories daily"

- Find a supporter who can be your accountability partner for your goal

Goal setting can be exciting and fun and can give you a specific plan for accomplishing a task that otherwise might seem difficult or even impossible. There are many goal setting programs available in book or online form. Learning how to set goals for your life will literally change your life for the positive.

TAKING ACTION

Now that you know what your goal is and how you will look, feel, and live when you hit that goal, it's time to take action. I'm a fan of Massive Action. One of my mentors, Tony Robbins, promotes massive action. This is taking action by immersing oneself in the task. You cannot lose significant weight by dabbling at weight loss. You must immerse yourself in the entire weight loss process as I've previously described. Small actions get small results. A common thing that I see among weight losers is that they do very well Monday through Friday evening. Then they eat more on Friday night, Saturday, and Sunday. They may not severely overeat, but they eat a higher amount of carbohydrates and calorie dense foods. The body can burn only two fuels. One is sugar and the other is fat. Our body prefers to use sugar as its primary fuel. When our diet is rich in moderate to high glycemic foods (those that convert to glucose readily) we will burn the sugar we need and convert the unused sugar into stored fat. When we restrict our calories below our daily needed calories then we dip back into our fat stores for the additional fuel. This fat is converted into ketone bodies which can be used for fuel. If we lower the amount of carbohydrates (sugar-based foods) in our diet and increase our protein intake, we can increase the amount of energy expended to process our food into fuel. We can then direct our body to preferentially burn stored fat, as long as our calorie intake is reduced. When people eat a reduced calorie diet Monday through Friday evening, they are appropriately working toward burning fat. It takes the body several days to burn off stored sugar and to then dip into the fat stores for energy. If a lower calorie, higher protein diet is started on Monday morning, then by Wednesday evening the body is converting over to increased fat burning. This takes about 72 hours of restricted calorie intake to occur. On Thursday and Friday, the dieter is in full fat burning mode. The problem starts when the increased food or carbs are taken in Friday night, Saturday, and Sunday. The body then converts back to burning sugar as its primary fuel source and makes fat out of any excess sugar calories. When Monday comes, the person is disappointed that they have lost no weight and feel like they've failed at this plan. This type of dieting is common and people can't understand why they are not losing weight. To lose consistent fat stores and weight, a reduced calorie plan with reduced higher glycemic carbohydrates must be carried out in a persistent manner. We must keep our body in fat burning mode day in and day out. This is the reason I have a problem with "cheat days" where a person will diet for 6 days a week and then eat what they want 1 day a week. This one day a week sets them back by at least 3 days of fat burning and weight loss. This becomes so frustrating for most people that they throw in the towel and go off of the program altogether.

Sustained action is mandatory when losing weight. In my clinic, I will assist patients to stay in the fat burning mode through great tasting higher protein snack meals, and, if needed, the use of appetite suppressing therapies using supplements or medications to control the craving for sugars and increased food volume. I let them know that they are at war against fat and the resistance to fat loss. Their body does not want to lose fat. We are designed to store fat as a survival mechanism. Even when our body chemistry goes awry or our genetics predispose us to store and hold fat and weight goes up to 350, 400, or even 500 pounds, our body resists fat loss. I have patients who have been in this very high weight range and with the loss of 20 to 30 pounds, their body and mind start to work to slow down the fat loss. Even with hundreds of pounds of extra fuel storage in the body, it is natural for an acute weight loss to cause changes in biochemical and hormonal processes and signals that tell our body we are starving. The body sends signals to the brain telling us to eat more. Hunger signals are magnified and our eating centers in the brain tell us to focus on higher calorie foods. It is mandatory to be able to break through our body's and mind's rebellion to weight loss. I use all means necessary to keep the patient on track and being able to interfere with these hunger and eating signals is important, especially in the first few weeks or months of the fat loss process. As weight continues to fall and the body and mind accept these new eating patterns and fuel supplies, the cravings and hunger signals do calm down. At this point, staying on plan and moving toward the initial goal is better tolerated. I didn't say easy. Any program that says weight loss can be easy is dishonest. A plan can be simple, but dropping excess fat is never easy. It's work.

CHAPTER 10
YOUR ACTION PLAN/TAKE MASSIVE ACTION NOW!

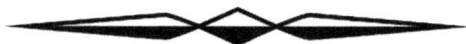

STEP ONE OF YOUR WORK—THE DIET

The right eating plan is necessary for any weight loss to occur. We call it a diet when we alter our food intake and change the pattern of food consumption. There are many people out there stating that you should never "diet". This is just marketing. We must change our eating pattern and our diet to lose weight and to keep it off. Calling it a "lifestyle change" instead of a "diet" is just semantics. Call it what you will, but I still call it a diet. Over my lifetime, I have seen so many diet plans and programs for weight loss that we would expect everyone to be skinny. Unfortunately, when it comes to weight loss and fat reduction, the great majority of people focus only on the eating. It's true that what we eat is critical to a healthy body, but remember as previously outlined, it is only one component of weight loss and long term weight maintenance. Remember that losing weight is not like treating a cold. We can't just focus on the problem with a short term solution such as the diet of the month.

Many scientific studies have been done to determine what the best dietary program is for losing weight. Many have concluded that a calorie is a calorie is a calorie. That is true in the lab where food substances are burned in a calorimeter to determine the calorie content of a food. In the body, however, different food substances are processed differently and result in varying calories that are available for energy. We know that a gram of carbohydrate and a gram of protein provide 4 calories of energy as determined by the calorimeter machine. Our body sees them differently and treats them differently. Simple carbohydrates are rapidly moved directly into the blood as glucose (sugar). More complex carbohydrates are just chains of glucose that are easily turned into individual sugar molecules in the body. A single step is needed to turn these into useable sugar for energy.

A gram of protein has 4 calories which is equal to a gram of carbohydrate, but the breakdown process is much more complex. Each protein is a combination of amino acids. When we eat protein, we first must break the larger protein down into individual amino acids, which are then converted by multiple pathways into glucose for use as fuel. These amino acid conversion reactions require many steps and expend energy for this conversion to sugar to take place. The process is also much slower than simply turning a chain of sugars into a single sugar. Therefore, our level of sugar in the blood doesn't rise as quickly with protein ingestion as it does with carbohydrate ingestion. There have been some short term studies that show that our body can do fine with protein and fat alone and that zero carbohydrates are needed for us to survive. Elimination of an entire food source is not necessary to lose weight and fat loss can be achieved with a mild rebalancing of carbohydrate and protein intake ratios.

Our body does not just burn one source of fuel at a time, but does have a preference to burn a higher amount of sugar than fat. It is not correct to think that we are either burning fat or sugar at one time. We can certainly adjust the ratio of fat to sugar burning in favor of more fat burning by increasing exercise, our metabolic rate, and by altering our diet. Reducing total calories will move us toward greater fat burning and reducing total carbohydrates will move us to burn additional fat. The dietary regimens that I prescribe are balanced with about 30–40% from protein, 40% from carbohydrate, and 20% from fat. The total daily calorie intake is reduced to a range from 900 to 1300 calories depending on which of the three programs that one is on. Special circumstances exist for each individual and, therefore, adjustments of calorie intake and ratios of carbs, fats, and proteins must also be adjusted. Cookie cutter programs where every person is treated the same, will work for a few and not for others. Treating obesity is much like treating high blood pressure. A single medication or treatment protocol will not work for every one and, in fact, would be dangerous. The bottom line on fat burning is that we must eat fewer total calories than we need in a day. The more lean tissue that we have in our body, the greater the percentage of fat our body is able to burn. Without going into the more technical aspects of fat burning versus sugar burning, suffice it to say that to burn off excess body fat we must use more calories than we take in. We can do this by eating less or using more. The best way to accomplish this is to do both.

You will hear about low fat diets, low carb diets, water diets, ketogenic diets, very low calorie diets, and on and on. The absolute best diet in the world for weight loss is the one that you can stay on. This has to do with tastes, lifestyle, work schedules, and complexity of food preparation. Staying focused and committed to a lower calorie eating plan is necessary for consistent weight loss. In my clinic, I have patients on one of my three eating plans, or on a commercial plan such as Weight Watchers, Jenny Craig, Nutri-system, or other similar program. The object is to be on a reduced calorie eating plan that you can stick with. You must temporarily eliminate certain foods like alcohol, high sugar candies and snack-foods, fried foods, and particular foods that you may find set off a desire for increased eating. It is unreasonable to think that we can lose any significant weight without changing our eating pattern, but every day I encounter someone who tries to lose weight and continue eating in the same manner that got them to their overweight situation. One gentleman, in particular, was struggling with weight loss, but claimed to be eating specifically what I had prescribed. On further questioning, he confessed to continuing drinking his 4 beers a day. Habits are hard to break. I have another patient who confessed to buying large volumes of candy at a time due to post-holiday sales. Easter candy was discounted 75% the day after the holiday and even though she was on a weight loss diet plan, she purchased a high volume of the candy. Of course, we all know what happened with the candy and her resultant non-weight loss. Find a diet that you can live with, but that lowers the calorie intake and also reduces simple sugars and carbohydrates. Avoiding excessive fat in food will also lower calories nicely. I also encourage an increase in protein intake. It is important to discuss diet changes that are significant enough to cause marked fat loss with your healthcare provider, especially if you have other medical conditions or take medications. Be honest with yourself, track you daily calorie consumption and take massive action on the first step toward thin.

STEP TWO OF YOUR WORK—ACTIVITY (EXERCISE)

When I start someone on a weight loss program, I tell them that weight is about what we eat, and inches, fitness, and our metabolism is about exercise. I see many people who want to lose weight, so they hit the gym regularly and hard. After a few weeks of soreness and sweat, they are disappointed by little, if any, weight loss. If they have not reduced their calorie intake and focused on a weight loss diet, they will improve fitness, but still be fat. As I said earlier, you cannot out train a bad diet. If my patient has not been on any exercise plan, I don't start them on one until I see a 10–15 pound weight loss. This allows them to stay focused on their food intake until they establish a new pattern. At this point, I prescribe a gradually increasing walking program or step tracking program. When they have lost 10–15 pounds, their energy and motivation levels climb and it's easy to start adding physical activity to the plan. If a person has already been on an exercise program when starting my program, I have them continue with their current level of working out. After their initial weight loss, I have them increase either their exercise time or intensity. Increase in exercise intensity or time should be very gradual and deliberate.

I have seen many people get so excited that they sign up for "boot camps" only to sustain an injury and see their entire weight loss plan come to a halt. Be patient with yourself when it comes to exercise. It's extremely easy to become injured if you are overweight and haven't been regularly active for a while—like years. I love all of the step and activity tracking devices. I wear a FitBit daily and have for some time. It becomes a habit to see how much activity we are getting in a day. Tracking steps and activity, makes goal setting in this area much easier. My initial goal was to get to 10,000 steps a day. This is approximately 5 miles for most people. It took a few months for me to get there, but now I never miss 10,000 steps. For me to get 10,000 steps daily, I have to get on a treadmill every day. Seeing patients in my office is only a mild activity level. Over time, my walking has increased in speed and distance. As each of us drops weight toward our lean healthy weight, the ability to exercise with greater intensity develops. As weight drops and our lower calorie eating becomes more of a habit, exercise becomes a great way to maintain our lower body weight as well as keep to fat tissue in healthy ranges. For those that did not play sports as a child or teenager, developing a habit of exercise can be difficult. I find that putting on my workout shorts and shoes is the most difficult thing I do each day. Once they're on, the workout is never a problem. Choose a time of day that works for you and get started today. Set a work out goal, even if it's 1000 steps a day. Get a tracking device and begin. The old saying is true, "the journey of 1000 miles begins with a single step".

Weight maintenance depends on our body's ability to keep lean muscle tissue in a high range and body fat tissue in a low range. Normal percentages of body fat for adult women range from 16% to 28% depending on age. The older we are, the more likely we are to keep more fat on board. This holds true for men, but the normal ranges of body fat for adult men are from 12% to 22%. Keeping lean muscle tissue in a good operational state, takes consistent exercise. Consistent exercise also decreases inflammation in the body. I test and follow blood inflammation markers in many of my patients and find that daily exercise is the single most important factor in clearing the blood and body of inflammation. Inflammation is the hallmark of most disease processes in the body. When patients decrease their workouts to 3 days a week of activity, I see inflammation levels move upward. We were made to move. Our low activity lifestyles lead to tissue and blood inflammation, oxidation of fats and particles in our blood, and a decrease in our ability to clear toxins from our blood and organs. When my patients see the direct positive effect of daily exercise on their blood and organ inflammation markers and tests, they become much more motivated to continue daily physical activity. Most of my patients cringe when I advise daily exercise. They've heard that 3 times weekly for 20–30 minutes is good. The fact is that the 3 times weekly level of exercise is good compared to none at all. Any level of exercise is better than none at all. The best level is 1 hour every day of some form of moderate physical activity. When you can get to this level, you will increase the length of your life and reduce the risks of heart disease, stroke, diabetes, cancer, and most other disorders. If all of my patients hit this goal, I'd have much more free time on my hands.

Get a partner to exercise with. It holds us accountable to showing up for the activity and it's more fun. Being able to spur each other on, promotes a gradual improvement in our fitness level. A little bit of competition drives us to be better each and every time we exercise. I have several patients that share daily data with me. They know how much activity I've gotten and how many calories I've eaten and I know the same details about them. We also send congratulatory notes and encouragement back and forth throughout the week. They claim that having their physician tracking them daily has made a major improvement in their motivation and consistency of effort. They also have celebrated extra weight loss when seeing me in the office. They no longer dread stepping on the doctors' scales. You must do whatever it takes to begin moving more. Studies on exercise and even mild increases in movement show dramatic long term positive effects on our health. Just standing instead of sitting uses more muscles and has been shown to burn more calories. We live in a time where it is possible to walk less than 300 steps a day due to modern conveniences. We have luxurious vehicles to ride in. There are elevators and escalators to move on. We have remote controls to turn things on or off without leaving a chair, and nearly every person working is linked in some way to a computer or smart device. Our forefathers and mothers had to walk, lift, bend, carry, and move about all day to accomplish tasks that we can now accomplish with the push of a button. Enjoy the great new technology, but get active, get moving, and get lean.

STEP THREE—GET CHECKED OUT/GET PROPER TREATMENT

If weight loss is not easy for you, welcome to my world. It's time to find out why. Find a physician who understands weight issues and obesity and is interested in working with you to treat this disease and to put it into remission. If your doctor just says to eat less and exercise more and gives you a diet sheet, it's time to look for a new doctor. The treatment begins with a thorough understanding of your history, your family history, current medical and surgical history, medication and substance usage, and details about your attempts to lose weight in the past. A general exam is important in looking for signs of insulin resistance, hormonal imbalances, and other potential causes for the weight accumulation. Blood tests that look at our blood fats and lipids, blood count, general organ and chemistry functions, and some hormones is important to uncover subtle causes of obesity.

Once this data is evaluated, a specific plan for each individual can be offered. This includes the diet and activity prescription, but in many cases also includes short term medications to adjust the body's abnormal functioning due to the excess fat and its deleterious effects. Each person is different. As a result, I have different medicines that I can use as tools to treat glucose metabolism, appetite, PCOS, carbohydrate sensitivity, insulin resistance, emotional eating, and addictive eating behaviors. Not everyone who is trying to lose weight requires a medication. However, I've found that the chronic yo-yo dieter has underlying medical and psychological issues that need to be addressed and treated.

Treatment medications can range from Metformin to make the body more sensitive to its own insulin to Saxenda which acts on receptors to reduce appetite, increase satiety, and improve glucose metabolism. Other prescription medications I use for obesity treatment include phentermine (Adipex), Diethylpropion, Bupropion, Topiramate, SSRI's, Zonisamide, Qsymia, Contrave, and Belvique. In some cases, combinations of certain medications will lead to marked improvement of the disorder and control several symptoms at the same time. Close monitoring of patients on medication must be done. Though generally safe, all of these medications can cause side effects and may have the potential to interact with a patient's other medications. A trained obesity physician will be able to work with each patient to customize a proper plan that treats the underlying condition and creates a consistent fat loss with the desired reduction in body weight and improvement in health markers. Just knowing that you are overweight is not enough. Getting a proper evaluation of the problem and a specific plan of treatment will end the years of frustration and recurring failed attempts at weight loss. It will still be hard work, but the effort will result in major weight reduction and an improvement in health.

STEP FOUR: CHANGE YOUR THINKING, THE PSYCHOLOGY OF WEIGHT LOSS

Part of our initial evaluation also includes a psychological survey so that the patient and I know if any cognitive and behavior issues are major components in their obesity disorder and have been roadblocks in their attempts to get lean. If a patient has a serious eating disorder of a psychiatric nature, then I refer them to a psychiatrist for specialized care of this problem. Most patients do not have these psychiatric disorders. I do find that nearly 75% of our patients struggle with at least 1–2 emotional eating factors. When the patient is aware of these factors and goes through our cognitive training process to modify their behavior, they are much more likely to be successful in their weight loss attempt and much more likely to keep the weight down in the future. Having the patient go through a cognitive re-training program and then discussing their discoveries with their monthly visits is extremely important. Knowing the why behind your eating will lead to the ability to change the how behind your eating. Figuring out emotional eating triggers and learning how to be aware of situations that set off the triggers will facilitate the ability to make changes in the eating behavior. If a person knows that they eat when they are anxious, then the ability to sense anxiety and be prepared with more positive and specific ways to deal with it will allow for a major reduction in calorie intake. Knowing that perfectionism is a psychological pattern that you have it, will allow you to break through problems with your dietary program when you have a bad day or eat a food that is not on your eating plan.

There are techniques and tools that can be used to slowly adjust our thinking and allow us to modify our behavior when it comes to eating. To be able to change our thinking, which will lead to new behaviors and new habits, is a "must" and can literally change our lives for the better. This modification in our thoughts and resultant actions will also allow for long term maintenance of a fit and lean body. I call this "Forever Thin". I use a validated program designed by Dr. John Sklare. This program allows each patient to evaluate why they eat the way they do and addresses specific psychological issues that are a part of the root cause of their obesity and yo-yo dieting. Once these issues are delineated, an online study program is provided to allow each weight loser to work on changing their thinking. The exercises are simple and can be fun. I like to think of this as learning to trick our brain rather than having our brain trick us. Being able to change the way we think, will lead to the ability to change our actions and the resultant habits that have made it difficult to lose weight and keep it off. Correcting our thinking about eating and food can lead to better eating decisions and marked control of overeating.

Patients do return to our clinic after having reached their goal weight on our program and then have regained some weight. I wish I could say that we cure obesity, but that would be unrealistic. The best I can say is that we can get people to their optimal weight and provide tools that can keep them in remission of obesity. However, since the disease still exists in their body, there is a natural tendency for the weight to return over time. Without exception, my patients tell me that the reason the weight returned was related to a major life stress. They were working on their eating behavior, exercising regularly, working on their psychology, and continuing medical treatment when indicated, but when the stress became overwhelming, the use of all the tools went out the window and the eating pattern that made them fat initially, came back. This is much like a smoker who has quit but starts smoking again or an alcoholic that is sober and starts drinking again in that the underlying disorder returns with a vengeance when our mental health is tested. A major financial crisis, or the death of a loved one, or the loss of a job or any perceived major stress will trigger an outbreak of the overeating disorder.

The body and brain's chemistry rapidly reverts back to its baseline status and hunger along with eating of high sugar and high fat foods begins. A level of vigilance is needed especially in times of stress. When stressful events or an increase in the level of day to day stress occurs, it is imperative that we realize what is happening to us and take extra precautions to avoid losing control of eating and regaining the unwanted weight. Being aware of how we feel, what stresses are working on us, and how to deal with them in a better way than overeating will become second nature if you think about it regularly and act on it. Creating new ways to deal with stress and understanding that overeating in response to stress will only create more stress as you will worry about the added pounds as they mount up. This is something that all of us can do. We can learn to think in different ways and learn to respond in different ways. New habits will develop over time that will allow us to stop using food as a drug to alleviate stress. When this is achieved, maintaining a healthy weight will be more about the mechanics of healthy eating and exercise and less of a mind game. Changing your thinking will literally change your life.

STEP FIVE: BE ACCOUNTABLE

We can be accountable to ourselves, but there is a built in tendency to let ourselves "off the hook". We create "rational lies" in our mind to justify our behavior. No person in their right mind would ever overeat to a state of poor health. I've never met a patient who set out to become fat or obese. I've never accidentally eaten anything either. My eating was always on purpose and any overeating that I've done was related to the many variables I've been talking about. We must be accountable to someone. It's difficult to be accountable to someone who is very close to us such as a spouse or parent or child. Even good friends tend to be too lenient on us when we go awry in our weight loss efforts. An accountability partner should be someone who is not directly vested in your future and your life. They should care about you and your outcome, but not be emotionally involved in the process you are undergoing.

A great accountability partner in a weight loss effort can be an acquaintance or colleague or a friend who might not be your best friend. Someone who also needs to lose weight can be a great accountability partner if they are as committed to getting lean as you are. Making a pact with each other regarding your caloric intake or your exercise regimen is necessary. Communicating regularly about your progress is essential. As an example, it works best if you commit to exercising together and setting the time and day in advance. Knowing that not showing up will leave the other person wondering about you and alone in the endeavor is a great motivator. Having a coach, trainer, or diet counselor, is a wonderful way to have someone hold you accountable. Yes, you may have to pay a few dollars for the service, but their experience and wisdom with weight loss and physical exercise can be invaluable.

Recently I asked a couple of my weight loss patients to become accountability partners with me. We communicate through the software app called "My Fitness Pal". This allows me to see their daily eating and activity success. They also see what I've done for the day and we can send messages back and forth encouraging each other. It helps to have someone watching and cheering you on especially on days that you have not hit your goals. I have benefitted dramatically by having these partners. I believe they have also seen benefits from knowing that I'm watching them. It's easy to set a goal. It's hard to keep the day to day focus on the goal and its achievement. We must keep our eye on the end result. Getting lost in just the day to day mini-goals and not seeing the way we will look and feel when we've achieved our weight loss goal, will end with us not reaching the finish line. Our accountability partners will cheer the loudest when we hit the desired weight and begin to live the life we want when we are at our peak health.

CHAPTER 11
FOREVER THIN: THE PAYOFF

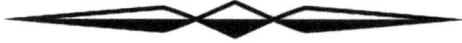

I ask my patients to sit quietly and picture in their mind how they will look when they are at their ideal weight. In the picture, I ask them to see what they will be able to do. Can they get on the floor with their children or grandchildren and play? Can they walk the dog without getting winded? Will they be able to wear the nice clothes that they've wanted to wear, but couldn't fit into? Will they be able to travel without difficulty? Will they be able to reduce medication for diabetes, high blood pressure, or high cholesterol? Will they add significant healthy years to their lives? All of these types of questions should be answered in the vision we want for ourselves and our lives. Better yet, why not paint the portrait just the way you want it. That way you will leave nothing to chance. You can create the life you want. Will it be easy? Of course not. It's not adult thinking to believe that you can reach your ideal state of health and look fantastic without paying a price. The price may be sore muscles. The price may include a growling stomach. The price may be giving up a dessert that you love. The price may include searching for a doctor that works with obesity and scheduling the check-up to see what may be causing your weight problems to be so difficult to solve. There will be a price to pay, but the price will be a bargain when compared to the benefits that you will have from putting obesity into remission.

A sleek sexy body that easily fits into the clothes you want to wear, is a great benefit. Having energy all day long is amazing. Eliminating sleep apnea, high blood sugars, high blood pressure, and high cholesterol is an incredible benefit. Being a positive example of health to your kids, your family, and your friends may inspire them to become healthier and that's a wonderful plus. Taking that long needed beach vacation and fitting into a swimsuit that complements your body instead of hiding it is a feeling we all want and can have when reaching our goal weight. Being more sexually attractive to our partner and having a greater sex drive is a benefit many patients get from reaching their optimal weight. Playing sports again or enjoying hiking or cycling again is a marvelous benefit. The world will feel different at your ideal weight. Possibilities that seemed unattainable will now seem possible to achieve. When you have a body that is thin and strong, other positive things will begin to happen in your life. Achieving a major goal such as reaching your ideal weight can set in motion momentum in other areas of your life. I have seen many patients who have reached their desired weight and have then developed a new relationship or found the person of their dreams. I've seen people that are now at their optimal weight achieve greater things in their work and careers including promotions, raises, and even starting their own business. What happens is that when we achieve a major goal such as losing all of our excess fat and reach a trim, healthy weight, we realize that anything is possible. We have beaten and learned to tame the one thing that has frustrated us for much of our lives. When we attain victory with respect to weight loss, then we know that we can work the process in any area of our lives. One success is likely to beget another. All success is found by using similar principles. Decide what you want. Set the goal. Take massive action in the direction of your goal. When obstacles occur (*Resistance*), work harder, smarter, and think better to overcome them. Review your progress regularly and make corrections in your direction so that you end up achieving your goal.

Losing weight and getting healthy is hard work. There is no magic involved. There is no special pill or training device or any other "cure" for this disorder. A systematized and consistent plan to change your life is required. Staying closely on your plan and tracking your progress is a must. Your life is well worth the effort. It's truly amazing to see the transformation of a person who has discovered their weight loss problem, taken action to control the problem, and beat the fat genes and condition to arrive at their ideal weight. Their smile becomes 3 times larger, their energy is 3 times greater, and their zest for life becomes unlimited. Through the journey to thin they have learned things about their mind and their body that they didn't realize before. They've learned that even though they had many failed attempts at losing and keeping weight off in the past, the ability to succeed was within them all along. They just needed the right tools and the entire formula for sustained long term weight loss and maintenance.

We all think we know the answer to weight loss, yet we leave out many aspects of the proper formula. Once the recipe is known and there is a true understanding of how to follow the recipe, the end product is a healthy, fit, lean body for life. I've coached thousands of patients to weight loss and I live my life working every day to maintain a lean, fit body. I mess up and get off track just like my patients, but am able to rapidly move back to proper eating and activity. My underlying genetics, biochemistry, hormone pattern, and stress eating patterns are like many of my patients. Given the chance, *Resistance* comes calling and attempts to send me off course toward a fat attack.

I understand what my patients are going through and I know when a person is serious and committed to getting lean and when they are just dabbling at weight loss. Dabbling in weight loss is a recipe for a failed attempt to get lean. Dabbling comes with the disease of excusitis. Excusitis is a condition where a person blames everything else on why they were unable to adhere to the plan I outlined. When a person gains weight on a dietary regimen designed specifically for their problem, they typically start feeding me excuses such as, I was stressed, or I was traveling, or I am allergic to all vegetables. The excuses are many times unbelievable and somewhat funny, though the problem of obesity is never a laughing matter. It's time to give up the excuses and be honest with yourself.

Look closely at your eating patterns. By knowing what foods you have trouble resisting and what foods you prefer to eat, you can get a reasonable idea of what the problem may be that has led to obesity. By opening up your mind to the possibility that you can take charge of what you eat and what you do no matter how many times you have tried, you will conquer the disorder once and for all. You can be the master of your destiny and live the life you have always dreamed of. Life is short and unless you decide today to take action to eliminate the fat and create a body that is lean, fit, strong, and healthy, you will continue to be frustrated each and every day. Make the decision. Take the action. Get the help. Find a partner to hold you accountable. Become who you really want to be and take the next step toward Living Lean, Living Long, and Living Life to the fullest.

Additional Information and Help

My practice focuses on helping patients get healthy by losing weight and getting more fit. Most medical practices focus on illness and the treatment and management of disease. By reducing excess body fat and increasing lean body mass, anyone can reduce the risk of disease and future medical problems. If you are struggling with weight loss and getting healthier, we'd love to assist you. For additional information on how you can become forever thin, check out our other resources.

Other Fat Doctor / Thin Doctor Series books by Dr. Oliver:

I Just Can't Lose Weight—Seven Reasons Why and How to Beat Them

Appetite Suppression

100 Points of Lite—Tips to Get and Stay Lean

WEBSITE:
FastClinicalWeightLoss.com

Join our community of health today. Email us at fatdoctorthindoctor@gmail.com to receive regular newsletters, updates, advice, training courses, and direct assistance to become forever thin.

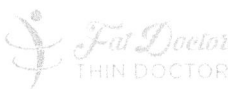

www.ingramcontent.com/pod-product-compliance
Lightning Source LLC
Chambersburg PA
CBHW050132280326
41933CB00010B/1340